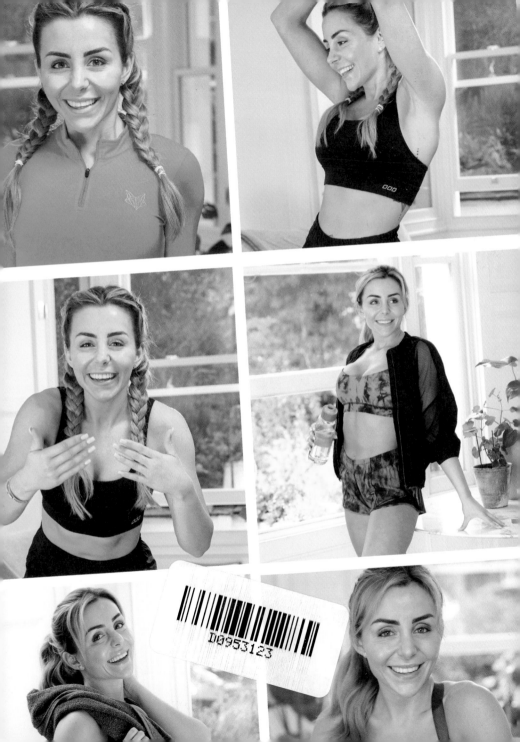

THE POCKET PT

Thorsons
An imprint of HarperCollins*Publishers*
1 London Bridge Street
London SE1 9GF

www.harpercollins.co.uk

First published by Thorsons 2021

10 9 8 7 6 5 4 3 2 1

Text © Courtney Black 2021
Photography © David Cummings 2021
Photographs on pages 18 and 21 courtesy of the author

Courtney Black asserts the moral right to be identified as the author of this work

Contributing writer: Becky Howard
Stylist: Sarah-Rose Harrison
Hair and make-up: Bella Campbell

A catalogue record of this book is available from the British Library

ISBN 978-0-00-844159-3

Printed and bound by GPS

MIX
Paper from
responsible sources
FSC™ C007454

COURTNEY BLACK

Thorsons

THE POCKET PT

No Gym. No Time. No Problem

CONTENTS

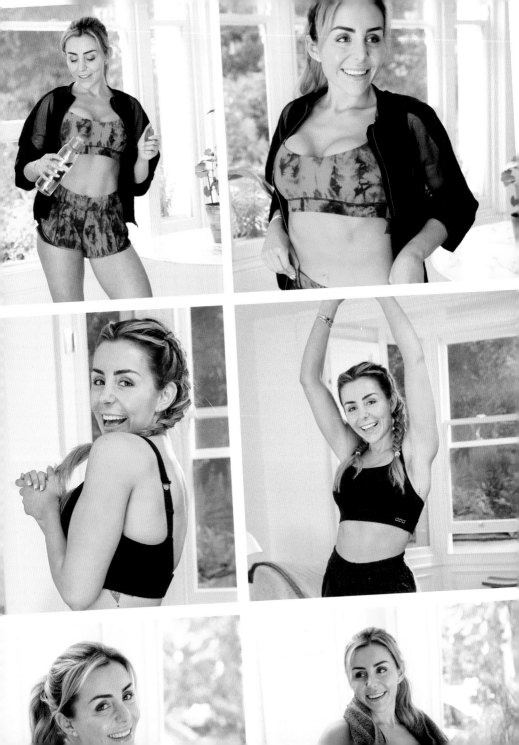

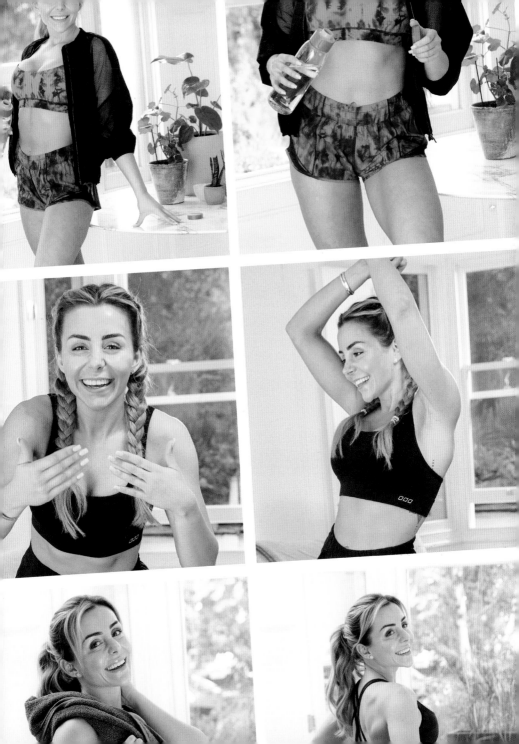

Introduction

Hi!

Firstly, I want to say a massive thank you to everyone who's picked up this book. You've made the first step in an amazing journey towards being a fitter, stronger, healthier and HAPPIER person all round.

I can't believe I've got a book, to be honest with you. Just a few years ago I was in such a bad place. I was doing my brain and my body real damage. I didn't eat properly, I exercised obsessively, I compared myself negatively with everyone else online. Basically, I was miserable. I lost who I really was in the empty search to try to be someone else.

Now, I'm a totally different person – happy, healthy and strong. But it took me a long time to get here, and I've learned loads of lessons along the way. I've learned that food is your friend, and fitness can be truly enjoyable, when it is part of a really positive lifestyle.

If you're sitting here thinking, there's no way that I'm going to ever think that, and there's no chance I could stick out a 28-day fitness plan, well, I'm here to tell you that you can. You can do this. Anyone can get fit and enjoy it – whether you're a total beginner, or whether you

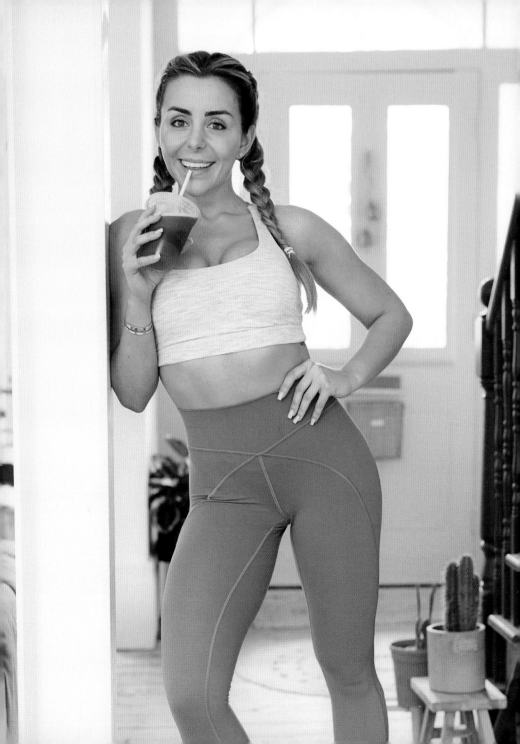

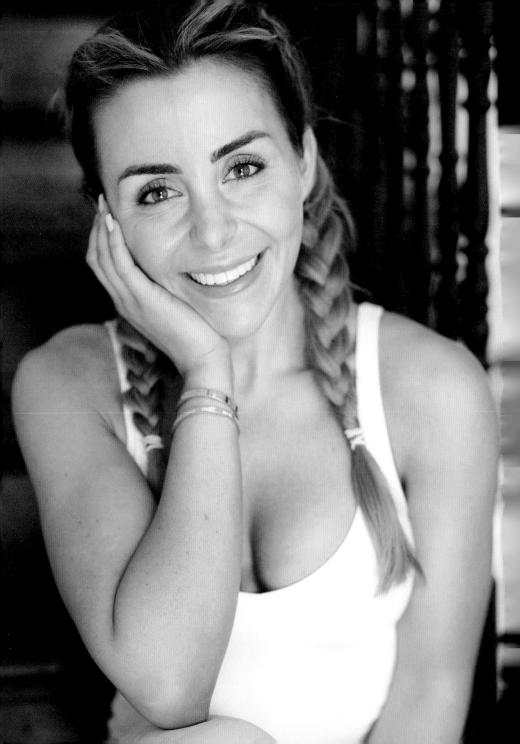

do it but really hate it! Don't be too hard on yourself. It's fine to be a beginner. You're making a start in the right direction and that's what counts.

I've made so many changes for the better in my life. In this book I'm going to share them with you, so you can see that it is possible to change your habits, and transform your life. I used to punish myself for not having the so-called 'perfect' body, and it made me miserable. This book isn't about punishment, it's about positivity.

I'll show you how to shift your mindset into a healthy place, where you can achieve your goals. We'll go through a 28-day workout plan, which will transform your attitude to fitness and leave you feeling better than ever before.

My promise to you is simple – you won't regret doing this. After four weeks working out with me, I swear it will feel amazing. You won't regret working hard to get yourself fitter and make your lifestyle more positive all round. You'll be a fitter, healthier, happier version of yourself and you'll love it.

I'll be here with you every step of the way babes. Let's go!

Love,
Courtney

PART ONE – MY STORY

A little performer

I'm a proper East End girl. I was born on 31 July, 1996, in the Royal London Hospital, Whitechapel. I've lived in the East End of London pretty much my whole life, first in Stepney Green, then in Bow. People say you're only a proper Cockney if you can hear the sound of Bow Bells, so I think I definitely qualify!

I'm the youngest in my family – my older sister Hadley was three when my mum, Colette, had me. I was a proper little performer from a really young age, confident and headstrong, putting on shows for my family. I'd sit them all down and make them watch me! But I've no idea where that part of me came from – no-one else in my family was like that at all.

My mum worked in soft furnishings, making curtains and blinds from home, where she had a little table with all her kit set up. My dad David worked in the theatre, but not as an actor. He worked behind the scenes, in set building, for the Royal Ballet at the Royal Opera House in Covent Garden. Although I was never interested in going to see opera or ballet, going to the theatre was a big part of my childhood. I went to see everything I could – *Les Misérables*, *Billy Elliot*, *The Lion King*. I found the experience of going to see those

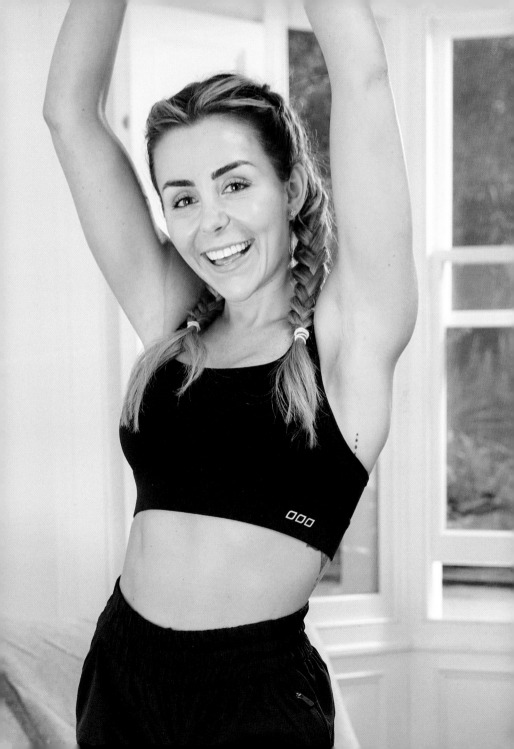

big West End shows totally magical. It felt as if I was stepping into a different world. It was amazing. I was a happy kid, in the main. When I was little, I was a real daddy's girl, and had a brilliant relationship with him. But, sadly, things changed for the worse.

I had so much energy as a little girl, so my mum enrolled me in weekend classes at the Italia Conti Academy of Theatre Arts. It's one of the UK's most famous performing arts schools and loads of its former students have gone on to be incredibly successful, like Naomi Campbell and Pixie Lott. Every Saturday, we'd walk together to the classes in Bow, and I'd spend hours doing ballet, tap – all sorts of dancing. I loved everything about it – it took me away from the normal world and I'd look forward to it all week. The uniform looked horrible – bright blue Lycra flares, with a tight blue and white top! – but it didn't matter. Those classes were my happy time. Even back then, though, I knew I wasn't good enough to be a professional dancer. I wasn't the best of the best. In the back of my mind I thought that maybe I could be a dance teacher, but there was no way I was going to put my whole career into dance. I didn't know what my future held, but I was always focused and driven to succeed. I didn't want to do something where I knew I wasn't quite good enough.

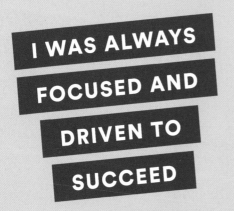

I WAS ALWAYS FOCUSED AND DRIVEN TO SUCCEED

Finding focus – but not friendship

At 11, I started secondary school, but not the local one to us in Bow. My mum wanted me to get my head down and study, so I went to a girls' convent school, St Ursula's Convent School, in Greenwich, south-east London. There were nuns in the school – though they didn't teach us! – and we had to go to church every week. It was pretty strict, too: no make-up allowed, no phones. Despite this, I'm really glad I went there, and if I had a daughter in the future, I'd definitely send her to the school. I think you get too distracted when you're around boys at school. When I was at St Ursula's, I just used to roll out of bed in the morning, get ready quickly and go to school to learn. I didn't stress about my appearance or anything like that. It was easier.

Having said that, I was a bit of a loner at school. I didn't have many friends, apart from two local girls who also went to St Ursula's, Harriet and Daisy. We didn't have class together, but I'd sit with them at lunch, even though we were really different. I used to pick Harriet up on what she was eating all the time – I'd bring in my salads, whereas they'd all be eating chips and junk food. My issues with food were just starting then – I'll tell you more about that in a bit.

Apart from Harriet and Daisy, for the first few years of secondary school I didn't really bond much with anyone else. I've always been super-focused, and strong-minded, like I say. I don't think most kids really understood me back then. I'd do my homework at lunchtime, which led to a few people

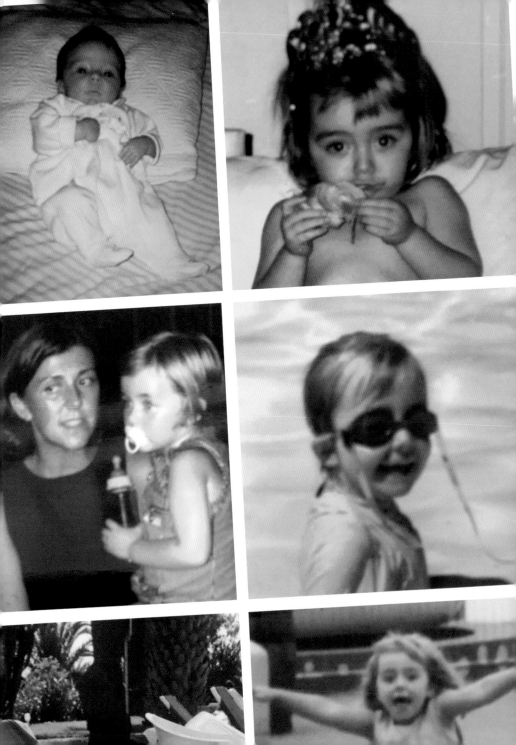

taking the piss and calling me a teacher's pet, but I didn't care – it meant that I had more time in the evenings to play computer games. Oh my God, I was obsessed with *The Sims*! I'd play it all the time, as well as another online game called *Stardoll*. You'd make your own doll, buy her clothes and go shopping – I was really into fashion, too – and I even made a magazine about it on Photoshop!

The most hilarious thing happened when I was about 14. I won a competition on *Stardoll*, and the prize was to meet a girl band called The Veronicas. Only thing was, I had no idea who they were, but the competition was supposed to be for their biggest fans! Me and my mum got taken in a taxi to central London for a proper day out and we were frantically googling them on the way. When we got there I had to interview them – it was so embarrassing. I'm sitting there with them, and they're saying to me, 'Oh, you know this song of course,' and I was like, 'Er, no?!' It was so funny.

My family shatters apart

My life changed totally when I was 13: my parents broke up. To me, an innocent kid, it came out of the blue, but looking back the signs had been there for a long time. My mum would cry a lot, and although she didn't tell us what was really going on, it was clear she was unhappy. I now know she was trying to keep their relationship together for us kids. It was a messy break-up; my dad would come round and they'd have huge rows.

Although I had been really close to my dad, strangely I wasn't that emotional when they split up. I was more upset for my mum, because she went through such a horrible time. My dad's family made it really difficult for her, turning on her, and it was so awful to see. Before that, both sides of my family had got along really well. Even my dad, who I'd been really close to, turned on me, too. I saw him a little bit after he moved out, but I felt like he hated me for being so close to my mum. He stopped making any effort with me or trying to keep our relationship going. I don't speak to my dad any more, now. It's sad, but he hasn't been a proper dad in years.

Luckily, my mum met another man a few years later, my stepdad Nick. Originally, I thought he was a bit weird. We were an all-female household, city girls from London. Nick was a fireman, from the Essex countryside, who was obsessed with fishing! Me and my sister originally thought he was a bit odd, but now I think he's the best person ever. I just love him. He was always great with us – even putting up with our teenage parties in the house – and he makes my mum so happy. They got married when I was 18, and have now moved out to Chelmsford, where he's from. It's amazing to see my mum, who's totally my best friend, with someone who really looks after her.

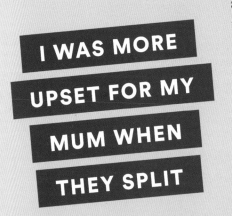

I WAS MORE UPSET FOR MY MUM WHEN THEY SPLIT

At the same time that my parents were splitting up, I was getting into dance in a big way. I'd left Italia Conti and started going to Latin and ballroom dancing classes three or four

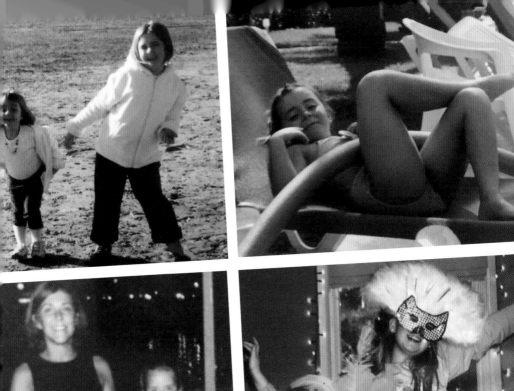
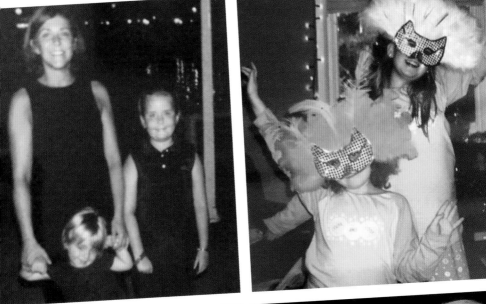
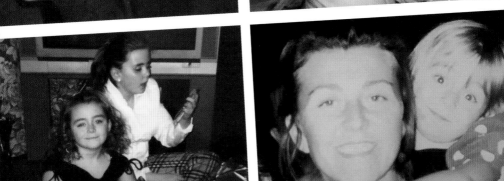

times a week – bless my mum, she took me everywhere! Not only to the classes but driving me up and down the country for competitions at the weekends, everywhere from Reading to Birmingham and Blackpool. She even made my costumes for me, because she was just such a good seamstress. Oh God, there was one costume I remember really well. It was a tight, clingy one made out of baby-pink Lycra! I had a bit of a tummy in it, which I'd become aware of, especially standing next to my friend Daisy, who looked like a stick in the same outfit. But despite my self-consciousness, I used to love the dancing, particularly the competitions. I took part in the Open Dance Championship at the world-famous Blackpool Dance Festival, which was such an amazing experience. The lights, the ballgowns, the make-up ... everyone is so prim and perfect. All the boys are in tuxedos. It's like something out of an old Hollywood film. You literally feel like a princess. It's just great. It's like a different world.

Food becomes the enemy

Around the time I was taking part in the Open Dance Championship, I started to develop an unhealthy relationship with food. Having to fit into those tight, clinging Latin dancing dresses made me more aware of my shape. As a little girl, I'd been a bit chubby, but I wasn't huge at all. However, in my early teens I got obsessed with dieting. I'd started watching the Victoria's Secret catwalk shows and, like I said, I'd got really into fashion, too. I wanted to look like

'Don't worry about failures, worry about the chances you miss when you don't even try.'

JACK CANFIELD

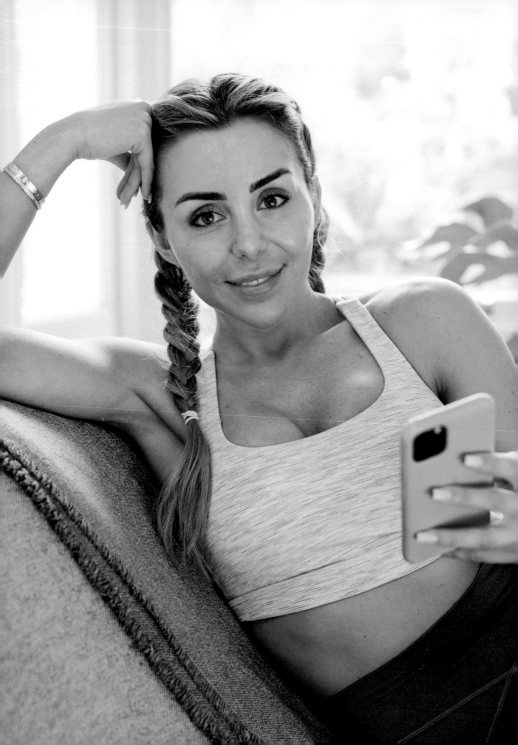

the models I watched strutting down the runway. I started comparing myself negatively to them, so I began to only eat 'healthy' cereal every day: for breakfast, lunch and dinner. I had a sweet tooth, I wanted to be skinny, so I thought it was a win-win, even though it was so bad for me. Looking back, I just think I was so stupid and uneducated. I had no idea how important food was in helping my body and brain function well. I just thought I had to eat a little bit to stay alive. I literally had no idea.

I didn't realise I had an eating disorder. I was just a girl who wanted to lose weight and look a certain way. Now, I wish young girls wouldn't compare themselves to models the way that I did. It needs to be drummed into young girls' heads that it's the models' job to make the clothes look good, and you shouldn't judge yourself by their standards. They're beautiful in a certain way, sure, but you're beautiful, too. So many girls think the way I used to – 'I must have the perfect life', 'I want to look like that and then my life will be perfect, too' – but it's total rubbish. No-one has the perfect life, and trying to look like someone else will only lead to misery.

A traumatic experience

Despite my terrible eating habits, I carried on doing ballroom and Latin dancing, getting skinnier and more unhealthy. I had a really bad experience, however, that put me off that world forever. I was 15 and I had a dance partner – let's call him Alex. We worked really well together and had lots of success. It's hard to find a good dance partner because you need someone you blend well with, who's a similar height to you, all of that. You stay round each other's houses before competitions, and you have to get along really well because you're with each other all the time. I was staying at his family's house one night before a competition when I got the shock of my life. I'd just finished in the shower when I spotted that he had set up a phone in the shower to video me. I was absolutely furious. I confronted him straightaway and he didn't even deny it. It was disgusting; his mum was appalled. I had to get the train on my own to our dance class in Reading, and tell all our teachers what had happened and that I wouldn't be dancing with him anymore.

THINGS GOT A LOT WORSE BEFORE THEY GOT BETTER

I felt more angry than anything else. If he'd managed to get the video out there, I can't imagine what would have happened to me, but luckily I'd been able to delete it. I felt really demotivated after that experience – obviously I wasn't going to dance with him anymore but I couldn't find another partner that I blended with as well. It felt like two years of dancing together, all that work, all that time and sacrifice, went down the drain because of what he did. After that, my interest in dancing just sort of faded away.

Exercise becomes an obsession

In place of dancing, I became obsessed with exercising in the gym, and my new life meant I could do that all the time. I'd left sixth-form college after a year because I just wanted to get into the workplace, earn money and be independent. I'd done two apprenticeships and then bagged a job in an accounts payable department at a company in Oval, south London. To be honest, I wanted that job mainly because there was a 24-hour gym in the basement underneath the office. I would get to the gym at 7am and go running on the treadmill for ages. Once I even got there at 5am, even though I didn't need to be in the office until 9am. I'd try to get all my work done before 12pm, then I'd go back to the gym for another session. I didn't take a proper lunch break or eat proper food. It was really bad. This extreme exercise really affected my work – I had no energy, I'd make mistakes all the time, then I'd nearly fall asleep on the train on the way back. I was really antisocial, too. I'd never go out with the rest of the team to work lunches, or out for events in the evening: I was worried about the food and drink that would be available, and wanted to make sure I could get up for the gym in the morning, so I'd get home, totally done in, and go to bed at 6pm.

It was no way to live – I was only 18 or 19, and I should have been having fun, enjoying my life. But things got a lot worse before they got better. Thanks to my eating disorder and extreme exercising, my body was craving calories and energy. I was desperate for sugar, so I started to buy chocolate bars just so I could chew them up and spit them out. It was awful. I was buying four or five a day, then hiding in the toilets at work to spit them out as I couldn't have anyone see me do this. I got so obsessed. I was really judgmental, not only with myself, but also of what everyone else was eating. I thought they had no self-control. It was such a messed-up attitude, but I was locked inside my obsession. I knew it wasn't right, though. Once I even filmed myself doing the chewing and spitting, to try to shock myself into stopping, but I still carried on.

I had such an unhealthy relationship with food – I literally saw it as the enemy and if I could find any way to eat less and get more energy, I would. I was eating all those fake foods – zero-calorie noodles, sweeteners and shit like that. I was putting so much crap into my body. I now know they're full of rubbish. The more of them you eat, the more food you crave. And it happened to me; the more I ate these zero-calorie things, the more I would crave sugar and calories. I'd then binge on rubbish later on. My body was crying out for proper food and nutrition, but I was in such a damaging cycle of behaviour back then.

It affected every part of my life. I'd started going out with a guy called Mitch after I met him on a rare night out. I was unhealthily skinny, and he'd try to help me by bringing round pick 'n' mix all the time – he knew I'd eat it and he was trying to help me put on weight. But I wasn't interested. We went on holiday to Turkey and it was a disaster. I was waking up at 5am, going to the gym and going to breakfast on my own. He got the hump with me and we had a blazing row, so

THE KEY
TO SUCCESS
IS TO FOCUS
ON GOALS,
NOT OBSTACLES

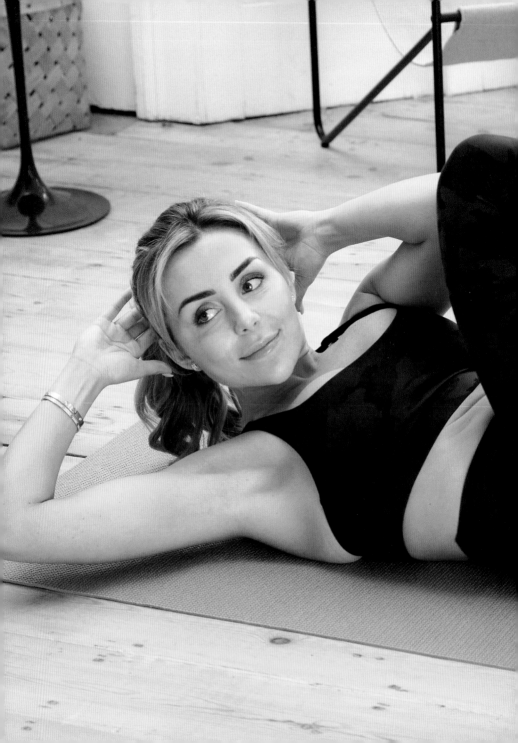

I got the plane home after just four days. I thought he was totally in the wrong – and he wasn't perfect, far from it – but now I think, poor bastard. We broke up not long after that.

Compare and despair

I was already on Instagram by this point, but now I look back at my early posts and I cringe. I'm so not that person anymore. It originally began as a little social thing for me and my friends, and I started off posting about fashion. It grew bit by bit, and I started posting more fitness stuff, but it was all about my appearance, basically. I'd look at celebrities, film stars and fitness people on Instagram, and compare myself really negatively. Why haven't I got the same body shape as them? Why doesn't my waist look like that? Why doesn't my nose look like this? And of course, when you post stuff on Instagram, you're making yourself look the best you can be, sucking in your belly, only posting the best photo ever, retouched, all of that. I built up some followers that way, but I was selling a lie, making myself look like the so-called perfect person. It made me totally on edge, because that's not who any of us are in real life. It was all 'look at me', all flashy and superficial, no substance. My followers didn't care that I was a funny, nice person, they just cared about my skin, my hair, my body. It wasn't real. But at the beginning, that attention is hypnotic. You love all the comments saying how amazing you look, but then you have to wake up the next morning and you don't look like the

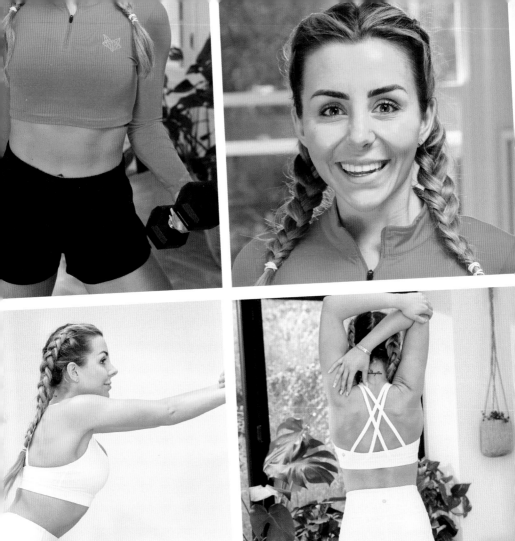
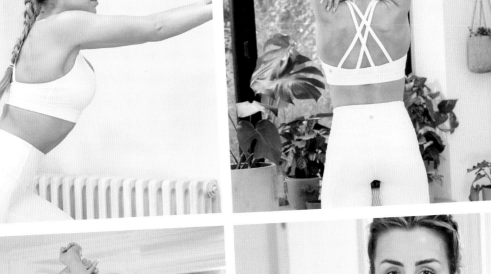
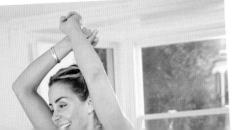
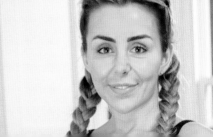

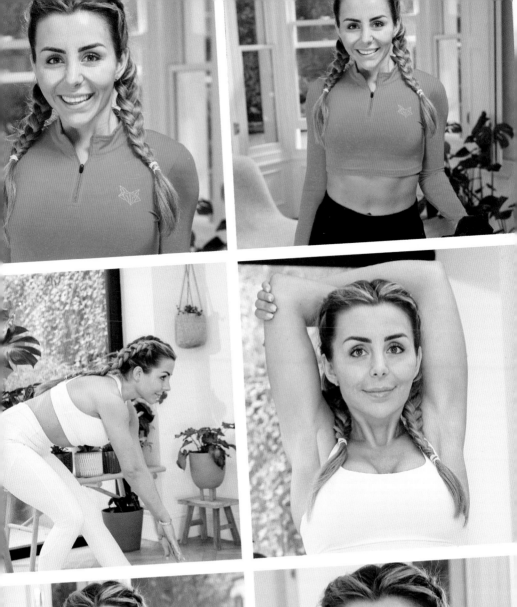
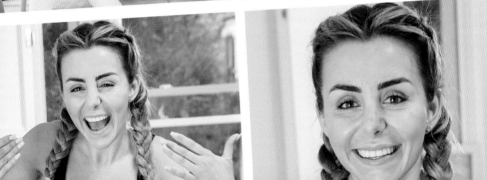

person you put up online, you feel really shit about yourself. It's a horrible feeling, when you try to sculpt yourself into something you're not.

Oh God, I was covered in fillers, too. At one point, when I was 19, I had them in my cheeks, chin, jaw, nose and lips. I had a package called the 'Kylie' done, which was based on Kylie Jenner's face. Everyone was obsessed with that look, and I fell into the trap of thinking it was normal. But that's not my face, that's not how it was designed. I wasn't supposed to look like that. My mum would tell me my lips were too big and so were my cheeks: I had high cheekbones already, so what was I doing, putting in fillers? I literally woke up one day, looked in the mirror and thought, 'I look awful.' The next day I got them taken out.

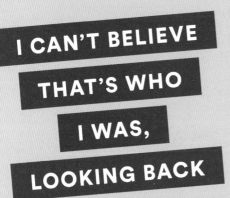

I CAN'T BELIEVE THAT'S WHO I WAS, LOOKING BACK

It was such a crazy thing to do. If I could say anything to my younger self – in fact, any girl thinking of getting fillers or any work done – it would be to really ask yourself why you want to do it. If it's because you're genuinely unhappy with something about your appearance and it's really affecting your life, then fine. But if it's because you want to look like someone else, don't do it. It's hard to push back if people around you are doing it – I know because I fell into that trap – but now I know you shouldn't ever try to look like someone else. You're you, you're unique, there's no-one else like you. That's what's special about us all.

My lowest point

Back when all this was going on, people were worried about me. They had noticed my exercise obsession, and that I hardly ate. The staff from the gym would call my office to ask if I was eating enough. My family used to pull me up on it, asking me at birthday dinners why I wasn't eating. My poor mum didn't know the half of it – I was hiding a lot from her because I was at work, or the gym, practically all the time. She was onto me, though, as she knew I wasn't looking after myself. But things got really bad when I went on a cruise round the Mediterranean with her and my stepdad. I didn't go out once for dinner because I didn't want to eat that late – I wouldn't eat past 3pm. I didn't go out on any of the day trips to amazing European cities because I was too tired. Instead, I spent my time in the gym. I became famous on the cruise – but only because all the crew knew me as the girl who obsessively ran on the treadmill.

I can't believe that's who I was, looking back. It has made me who I am today, but still, at the time, it made me so miserable. I had practically no social life – I stopped going to family birthdays and I wouldn't go to parties with friends, because I was so worried about the food and obsessed with getting up early the next morning. I was rude, exhausted and had totally lost my sense of humour. I wasn't myself. People couldn't get through to me, to make me see that I was too skinny, that I wasn't looking after myself. I didn't want to hear it. Things have changed so much since then, but it

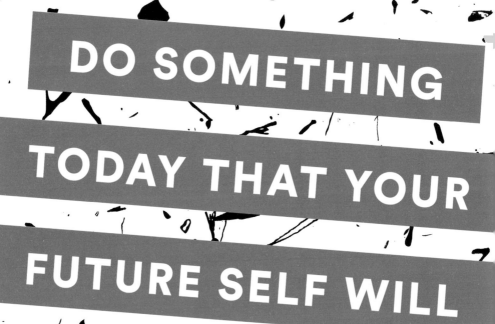

didn't happen overnight. It's been such a long journey.

Things started to change a bit for the better when I left my job to be a full-time personal trainer (PT). I'd already gone on a part-time course to learn more about working out in the gym, though to be honest my motivation then was about looking good. But I really enjoyed the course, and learning more about food and fitness. It was the first step into my new life. In contrast to the PT course, I hated my job in accounts payable. I couldn't stand working in an office; it was so depressing and stuffy. There weren't even any windows in there! I'd spend my spare time writing diet and fitness plans, then race back from the office in the evening to start doing PT sessions in the evening. It was insane, I was working 10–14 hours a day, but I loved running the sessions.

Eventually, I realised I wasn't going to excel in my life by staying in the office job. I had to make the move now. So, I quit. I knew it was the right thing to do – I lived at home, so luckily I didn't need to pay any rent. If things didn't work out with the PT thing, I could just get another office job at any time, but I was determined to make my new career work. I couldn't have imagined then how it would totally change everything in my life for the better.

More information about body image and eating disorders can be accessed via Beat, the UK's eating disorder charity: beateatingdisorders.org.uk.

PART TWO – YOU CAN CHANGE YOUR MINDSET

Opening up about my issues

By the time I was working full time as a PT, I had started to turn the corner. I'd put on a bit of weight, and was starting to learn more about good nutrition and lifestyle, especially from my friends at the gym. I was around people that I was having fun with, we were all like-minded, and they had my best interests at heart. But even though I was eating a bit more, and going out for the occasional team lunch, I was still doing the chewing and spitting thing. My eating disorder still had its iron grip over me.

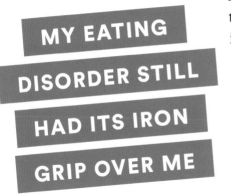

MY EATING DISORDER STILL HAD ITS IRON GRIP OVER ME

So far, I'd kept it a secret from everyone around me. I was embarrassed about it. But like I said, my mum was onto me, and she was so worried. Eventually, I told my mum what was going on. I had to, though, as she'd caught me doing it at home one evening when she spotted some chocolate was missing from the cupboard. Obviously, I was mortified. She wasn't angry; she was more shocked than anything else. The look on her face when she realised I was chewing and spitting out my food was pure confusion. 'What are you doing?' she asked me. I didn't really have an answer for her. I knew how bad it was, but this was the wake-up call I needed to make me think, I've got to knock this on the head somehow.

Although my mum knew, I didn't tell anyone else for a long time. If I'm being honest, it took years for me to learn how to eat healthily, and to be truthfully happy about my relationship with food. It's such a slow process, getting out of an eating disorder – don't let anyone tell you it's an easy thing to fix. A lot of it I put down to getting older and educating myself about food. I've always loved learning, so I got into researching nutrition online, through Instagram and YouTube – there are so many great resources out there – and I would follow people like Joe Wicks, Clean Eating Alice, London Muscle and US stars like Paige Hathaway. They all looked really strong and healthy, and I soon learned that you get like that by fuelling your body with the right foods, not by denying yourself.

Food becomes my friend

For me, I think the biggest change started to happen when I realised I didn't have to stop eating. I was following this ridiculous 'rule' that I couldn't eat after a certain time in the afternoon. But all that would happen to me was that I'd wake up starving in the middle of the night. My body desperately needed the food I was denying it. The gradual realisation that I was doing my body harm was a huge thing for me. I learned so much, too, from being around people I knew at the gym. I had a great teacher, called Josh, who was quite life-changing. He really helped me out when I was doing that PT course. He pointed out that because I was training, I needed more food than most people, not less. I was opening up my mind, taking all this in.

I started to eat more, and eventually I got to a good place, where I understood that going down the road of calorie restriction and fasting when you see food as the enemy is just crap. You always need energy, no matter what you're doing – whether you're in the gym, at work or sleeping. Food is amazing, and now I absolutely love cooking. I'm eating more than ever, but I'm eating really well. I've learned there are so many ways you can eat healthily.

I can't underestimate the huge impact this has had on all parts of my life. So many of the choices I made, at every single moment, were down to restricting my access to food. For example, I'd not go out for dinner because I wouldn't eat – I'd think, what's the point? Or I'd go out for dinner and not drink the wine because I was worried about the calories. Or my friend Georgia would invite me over for a Sunday roast and I'd say, 'Nah, I can't eat that.' Most of the time, I'd just end up staying in on my own. Restriction for me was such a big thing, but it made me feel shit, in every single way. It made me turn away from life, and set me on a downward spiral.

But this isn't who I am now. Not long ago, I went to a fitness camp in Thailand with a friend of mine. We had an amazing time and one of the best things for me was trying all the different Thai foods. God, I really loved the pad Thai and coconut mango sticky rice! The trip was incredible, such a good experience, and something that I never would have done before (or, if I had, I wouldn't have eaten the food, I'd have just stayed on the sunlounger all day). Now I was going out on boats, on day trips, exploring the islands, eating amazing food. I was so proud of myself for that.

Making fitness life-affirming

Changing my attitude to food went hand-in-hand with shifting my attitude to fitness, too. Like I said, I used to see it as just about being as skinny as possible, and basically like a punishment for eating. So, for example, if I'd eaten a sandwich, I'd think, right, that's 500 calories, and now I've got to run to get rid of that 500 calories. Now I know that you don't need to get rid of the food you're eating; you need it, babes! Your body needs food to stay healthy. Fitness is great, it can make you feel amazing, but only if you use it in the right way. You should exercise because you want to improve and maintain your health, because it makes you happy and makes a positive impact on your life.

But that wasn't the way I used to train. I was just, run, run, run, run, and a bit of abs. Cardio was my life. I didn't do any strength training, as I just wanted to be thin. Stupidly, I used to see training as a way of offsetting a binge at the weekend, too. I was so wrong. In fact, when I overtrained, I did my body damage. Now I know that exercising too much can actually cause you to put on weight, because your body goes into a state of overdrive. But gradually, I started using weights, I developed a bit of muscle definition, I got stronger. I learned that rest days are absolutely essential for keeping your body in the best state possible. The most important thing is to listen to your body. Now, I set my intent, I plan my workouts, I make sure I rest and I listen to what my body needs.

This has made me a better trainer over the years, too. At

the beginning of my PT career, I was still dealing with my own issues, and my approach was just to help people look good. Clients would tell me, 'I want to lose weight' and 'I want to look like so-and-so', and I'd be like, 'Okay, so do this, follow this exercise programme.' Now, I want to know how and why clients feel like that. The way you feel about how you look is not just about what you look like; it's about your emotional and mental attitude towards yourself. If you just train to look better, you're never going to get away from that negative attitude.

Learning to open up emotionally

It's an incredibly emotional job, being someone's personal trainer. I discovered that over time. You have to learn to relate to people and understand their psychology. At the beginning of my career, I was so locked into my own dysfunctional relationship with food, I didn't realise that many other people have a negative relationship with food, too. I remember one client in particular: I asked her to be honest about her problem with secret eating, and she burst into tears of relief, saying, 'No-one's ever talked to me about that before.' And this wasn't just one person – so many clients had other issues with food, too. There were girls who were binge eating, going to the supermarket, spending £15 on junk food, scoffing it all and making themselves sick. I realised it was such a sensitive subject for so many people, and that shame was a big part of it.

'IF YOU DON'T LIKE SOMETHING, CHANGE IT. IF YOU CAN'T CHANGE IT, CHANGE YOUR ATTITUDE.'

MAYA ANGELOU

When people opened up to me, it helped them, and it helped me, too. It's made me a more compassionate and empathetic person. For example, I used to not understand at all when people said they had an addiction to food. I was really judgmental of people who overate, thinking, well, why don't they just stop? I didn't get it at all; I thought it was just an excuse. But coming to terms with my own issues and then being around people who were really struggling with their own issues has made me a nicer person. I'm now 100 per cent a better trainer, a more understanding person. It's opened my eyes, made me a better listener and more mature. It makes me really happy when people open up to me, because it's an important first step in making a change. The whole thing for me now is about positivity, not punishment.

Making Instagram inspiring

Along the way, I changed my social media presence, too. I'd had enough of my posey Instagram profile. It wasn't getting me anywhere, and I knew people followed me just because I looked good. But like I said, it wasn't the real me and I was always on edge knowing that the image I was portraying online wasn't sending out the right message. I wanted to be a coach, to be an inspiring person, not the sort of person who causes others to develop eating disorders. I went through such an ordeal myself, and I knew I wasn't really helping anyone with my Instagram as it was.

So, I stopped being so self-absorbed. I stopped being obsessed with finding the 'perfect' angle to show off my exercises. I stopped sucking in my belly in pictures. Instead, I would post videos that showed me as I was when I was working out: panting, bending over with stomach rolls, doing burpees with my belly out. Initially, it was so nerve-wracking. I thought people would hate it, and criticise the way I looked. But then I realised – I don't care, let them unfollow me! If they are that shallow, then who cares? So I did it and it felt amazing. It was so rewarding to hear back from people that I'd inspired them, and it felt a million times better than any compliment about my looks. When you know you've made a difference – that's the most important thing.

One of the best lessons I've learned in the past few years is how to be comfortable in my own skin, and love my flaws. It's a breath of fresh air! It makes me so much happier and carefree. Always comparing myself negatively with other people was pointless, and I came to realise that we're all different, we've got different genes inside us that make us this way. Some of us are tall and leggy, some can run really fast, some can lift heavier weights more easily. It's just the way it is. You get so unhappy if you're constantly putting yourself down. I know I did.

Now I want my Instagram to make people feel good. I want them to feel like I'm their friend, that I'm encouraging them, making them feel better about themselves: I want people to feel amazing about themselves. I don't want them to feel like I'm putting them down, making them feel like crap because they can't relate. I'm there to help them, and encourage them to take home a positive message about food and fitness.

Not long ago I was on the phone chatting to my mum, having a massively emotional conversation about things. Actually, I'll be honest – I was crying, telling her that for the first time ever, I actually feel so, genuinely, happy. I feel like I'm being who I really am and I'm so content. Every single person who knows me has picked up on how much I've changed, and they're right. I just enjoy life now. I'm not ashamed of who I am. I'm being true to myself. I've gone through it, I've learned so much and now I want to pass that on, to you.

My life lessons

Okay, I know I'm still young, and I've got so much more to learn about life. But when I think about all the tough times I've gone through, all the shit I've done to myself, and all the incredible things I've learned from training people, it's taught me a lot. I've come out of it stronger and with a bit of wisdom under my belt.

For me, these life lessons are just really simple things to remember when you're trying to shift your own mindset from a place of negativity into a place of positivity. It isn't easy, I know, but you've got to believe that it is achievable, because it is! Start telling yourself these little mantras every day and, bit by bit, you'll find you start to develop a new attitude towards yourself. Starting a new fitness plan takes focus and dedication, and the reason a lot of people don't stick with it is because their mental attitude is tuned to negative.

1. We all start from somewhere

This is so important to remember whenever you start anything new – you'll always find it difficult at first. Always! Every single day I get messages from people on Instagram, saying, 'Why am I finding these workouts so hard? Why are you jumping about whereas I'm panting on the floor, feeling like I've got no energy?' It's because I've been doing them for years, but I wasn't always like this. I've got fitter gradually and built it up over time. It's also the same when it comes to developing my healthy mindset. I had slip-ups when I was overcoming my eating disorder – it was really hard. I just had to remember that it's fine to have a slip-up, tomorrow is another day. Just keep going, and don't let it put you off carrying on down the right path.

It's okay to be a beginner. Remember that. We're all too hard on ourselves, beating ourselves up saying, 'Why can't I do this? I'm crap!' But every single day you'll improve a little bit, and in a month's time you'll be able to do something new. So yes, you might feel like a total newbie, but take a step back and do it at your own pace. Rome wasn't built in a day. You'll notice an improvement if you push through it. Come back tomorrow. Don't quit!

2. What doesn't challenge you doesn't change you

This is another great one to remember when you're finding it hard to get going on a new fitness plan. They're supposed to be hard, so it's okay to find it difficult. It doesn't mean you're rubbish, just that it's a challenge. Think of it like this:

GREAT THINGS

NEVER

COME FROM

COMFORT ZONES

it's really nice to go on a walk every day, but that's not going to change your fitness as much as a really intense 30-minute workout will. Why? Because it's easy! Things that are easy aren't pushing you out of your comfort zone. You might feel battered at the end of the workout, but that's because you're making a change to your body, not because you're crap. In the long run you will feel so much better. I promise!

There are mental challenges, for sure, in getting out of negative habits that feel easy. Just like my chewing and spitting thing. It was so, so hard for me to break that, and it took time, but what motivated me was knowing that in the long run it would benefit me hugely. I knew it was for the best. So when you're finding the new fitness plan challenging, and just want to quit and lie down on the sofa, keep reminding yourself why you're doing it. You will notice a difference, you will get fitter, you will feel so much better. You have to just accept the challenge and go with it.

3. Food is your friend

Your body needs good food. I can't say this enough – food is NOT the enemy. It is your friend. Good food nourishes you in every sense of the word, and it is so important that you feed yourself well. Food isn't going to damage you unless you're overeating, or just eating total junk. Your body needs to burn calories every second of the day, so you need to nourish yourself with really healthy meals. Especially if you're training, you need more food than ever before. You've got to be nice to yourself, caring for your body by feeding it the food it needs, when it needs it.

Since I changed my mindset about food and started cooking and eating better, it's transformed my life. I'm just so much happier. I've got more energy, which makes me a nicer person. I love my body, too, and not just because I look a certain way, but because I'm so proud of all the things it can do. Having more energy means I can enjoy my life more, socialise and have fun. It all goes hand in hand. I was afraid of food before, but now I know it's so important to live well. Tell yourself that, enjoy your food, cook tasty meals and replenish your body before and after training.

4. Self-discipline leads to success

I read an amazing book called *No Excuses!: The Power of Self-Discipline*, by Brian Tracy, and it really inspired me. It's essentially all about how you shouldn't wait for luck, or chance, to bring you success – you can achieve it yourself by being self-disciplined about your own choices. If you don't put yourself or, for example, your business, first, then you're not prioritising your success.

So, for example, I was out with my friend on a Saturday night, and she wanted to stay out for a few more drinks. I could have easily said yes, but I had loads of things I wanted to do the next day and I knew I would have felt crap and not done them if I'd stayed out. So, I went home. I put myself first. Self-discipline is basically knowing what you need to do to get ahead in whatever it is you want to achieve, and doing it.

When you're starting my plan, put yourself first. Remember what you want to achieve, then plan your life around that. Get up a little bit earlier, don't spend so long on social media, tell your friends you're going to start a fitness plan so they can encourage you – whatever it is you need to do to make it work. You're not punishing yourself, you're giving yourself something amazingly beneficial. It's a gift.

5. You are a warrior

I just love this saying! It's so relevant to all of us. Because we all fight our own battles through life, like I fought my eating disorder. Everyone is always battling something – it could be low self-esteem, it could be illness, it could be difficult relationships, it could be anything. You never know what other people are going through and what their story is, so we should all celebrate that we're all pushing our way through things like the warriors we are.

It's also a reminder not to give up. I still sometimes struggle with wanting to do the easy thing, but I'll tell myself, 'Come on, Court!' I want to be a warrior, I want to boost myself up and remind myself what I'm capable of. You are a warrior, too, and never forget it.

All these sayings have meant so much to me, because I've fought hard to learn them. They weren't just hashtag inspo I read on Instagram, they're all truths that have changed my life, my attitude and my health for the better. I'm going to keep referring back to them – especially once we get going on the workouts – because I know they're gonna help you. You need to not be too hard on yourself if you're a beginner when it comes to exercise, but you also need to know that it's not going to be the easiest path: you need to make sure you feed yourself well, so that you're in the best physical place to smash your workouts; you need to have a big dose of willpower, to keep going through those workouts, those days when it feels hard; and, finally, you need to know that you are capable of anything, that you are a warrior. So I'm here to remind you, with my life lessons, that you've got this.

PART THREE – LET'S GET STARTED!

Okay, so I've shared with you the intense journey I've been on, and the life-changing lessons I've learned. Now it's your turn to start on your own journey with me by your side. I'm going to take you through the best 28-day fitness plan ever, one you can do from your very own living room, and we're going to do it together. Whether you're a total newbie to exercise or not, it doesn't matter. I know you can do it!

This section is all about getting in the right place – emotionally, mentally and physically – to start my plan. I want you to be in the best possible headspace so that when we start, you've got the right attitude and a positive mindset to succeed.

So many people start on a huge new fitness plan without preparing and thinking about it, and then they're surprised when it doesn't work for them, or they lose focus and quit. That's not going to happen with my plan, because I'm going to get you ready and raring to go. There's a famous saying that 'if you fail to prepare, you prepare to fail', and we're not gonna fail!

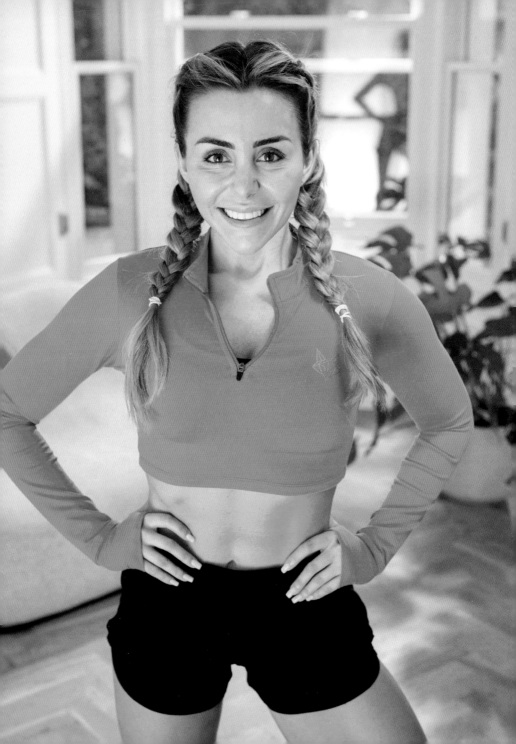

1. No gym, no problem!

Now, I've got a confession to make: I used to think you couldn't do a decent workout at home. I'm happy to admit that I was totally wrong! But let me tell you why I thought that.

Before the coronavirus lockdown in 2020, I'd never done a PT session at home in my life. I turned my nose up at it a bit, to be honest. I'd tried to do them a few times before and it hadn't really worked for me. I found it so demotivating to be at home. As you know, I was a total gym addict – I would do anything to train in a gym. Even when I went on holiday once to Nerja, in Spain, I would walk an hour in each direction every day just so I could pay €30 to train in a gym! It was madness – three hours out of each day on holiday just for that. Imagine!

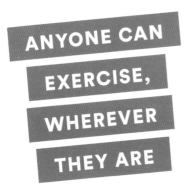

ANYONE CAN EXERCISE, WHEREVER THEY ARE

I didn't think I'd get the results I wanted at home. I didn't think you could achieve proper fitness goals without having all the gym kit and equipment around you. So I think I had the wrong attitude right at the start. But, I soon discovered that it doesn't matter where you exercise: anyone can exercise, wherever they are. Obviously, once lockdown happened, I couldn't get to the gym, couldn't get out, couldn't see my clients – I had to totally change the way I worked out. I started running daily live workouts from my small flat on my Instagram, and they changed my life!

It felt revolutionary to me. I could put my tunes on as loud as I liked, to get in the mood (no headphones needed). I could sweat as much as I wanted and not worry about looking weird (if I wasn't on Insta, I would have stripped down to my knickers – so you can do that!). You can nip to the loo for a wee if you need to without having to take all your stuff with you. I even used to think I'd get too hot in my apartment – well, all I needed to do was open the window! Best of all, you can give it your all for the entire time without having to travel anywhere and take more time out of your day to fit the workout in.

Everything about working out from home has been brilliant, and it totally changed my mind about it. I loved doing it, I loved connecting with my followers this way, and it was an amazing experience.

It showed me that although gyms are great – and I'm never not going to love my gym sessions – you can achieve just as good results from your own space. And you don't need a massive house, or a separate room to do your workout in – you just need to make a few preparations to make it work.

How to get your home workout-ready

- It's worth investing in a yoga or workout mat so you're not sliding all over the place when you're doing the floor exercises. A towel is nowhere near as good!

- Get some free weights, otherwise known as dumbbells! It would be best to get two different sets, with heavier ones that are a bit more challenging for when you're doing multiple reps. I can't recommend

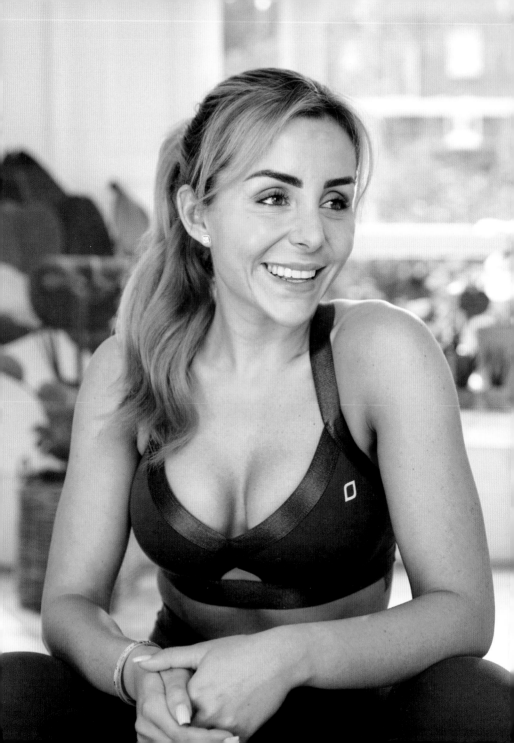

an ideal individual weight for you, as it really depends on your fitness and strength levels, but a basic guide for what you could invest in for your level of fitness is:

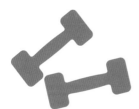

BEGINNER – I would recommend 2-6kg
INTERMEDIATE – I would recommend 5-10kg
ADVANCED – I would recommend 5-12kg

(You will find certain exercises too difficult using 12kg dumbbells, so read the guide that comes with the weights before deciding what weight to purchase.)

- Clear some space for your workout. You don't need a massive room, just move tables, chairs, boxes – whatever is in the way – to make sure you can put your mat down in a clear space and move your body around freely.

- Load up your phone with a brilliant workout playlist of your favourite tunes …

- … but put your phone on flight mode during the workout so you don't get distracted by notifications!

- Have a towel and a big bottle or glass of water ready before you get started, so you don't have to stop halfway through to get a drink.

Boom! That's it. Your home is now a gym.

2. You can find the time

One of the biggest excuses I often hear for not exercising is, 'Courtney, I don't have time to exercise, I'm too busy!' I hope this doesn't sound too harsh, but ... that's rubbish, babes! You do have the time. Everyone has 30 minutes in their day that they can give over to exercise – everyone.

Think about what you could save 30 minutes from every day. In the morning, you might be the sort of person who makes a really lavish breakfast every day – well, make something quick like porridge! You might spend ages in the shower, or deciding what to wear – get your outfit ready the night before. Rather than spending ages curling your hair every morning, tie it up in a ponytail and save that time. If you're working from home and take a full lunch hour to watch some telly, well, don't! Get a training session in before you eat lunch and you'll fit it into that hour, no problem – and what's more, you'll be set up for an amazingly energised afternoon. I used to find doing a workout just before lunch used to wake me up. In the evening, watch one less telly programme, and there you go, you've immediately got back that 30 minutes to do a workout.

Another super-easy way to grab back the time to work out is to think about your social media usage. Phones can now tell you how long you spend on them each day, and I bet that you can steal back at least 30 minutes from your time spent on social. Don't think of it as a punishment ... 'Oh, I would have a better time scrolling my Insta feeds' – no, you wouldn't! Carving out the time in the day to work out is a gift you can give to yourself, and it doesn't cost anything.

When's the best time to work out?

There is no ideal time to do your workout. It doesn't matter when you train, in terms of results, just that you DO train! There's so much misinformation out there about the 'right' time of day, and it's all rubbish. You're doing the same amount of work whether you do it first thing in the morning or last thing at night.

The biggest question you need to ask yourself is when suits you best. If you're like me – a total early bird who gets really tired in the evening – then do your workout first thing. I've always woken up pretty early in the morning and felt good, so this is perfect for me. If you're also an early bird, just have your quick coffee or whatever, then smash out your workout. You feel so good once you've done that, and then you don't worry about fitting in your exercise for the rest of the day.

I get a lot of questions on Instagram from people worried that they're not doing their workouts at the same time as I do. But there is no 'better' solution – the time I exercise is just the time that works for me. Honestly, by about 3pm I'm fading, so mornings are ideal! Have a think about your normal body clock, where your energy levels normally peak and fade, and you'll be able to work out pretty easily which time of day would suit you best.

How to work out when to work out

Don't worry if you can't think immediately which time would suit you for working out, especially if you're new to exercise. I've put together a few questions you can ask yourself to quickly figure out what might be the best time of day for you.

- Do you regularly have to work late? – work out in the morning

- Do you have a busy social life? – work out in the morning

- Do you find you wake up easily without an alarm? – work out in the morning

- Are you able to take a full lunch hour? – work out just before lunch

- Do you find you feel sluggish in the afternoons? – work out just before lunch

- Do you already have to get up early in the morning for work or kids? – work out in the evening

- Do you find it really hard to get up in the morning? – work out in the evening

- Do you get bored in the evening and end up snacking? – work out in the evening

How to make it stick

Plan, plan, plan! Once you've decided when to work out each day, put it in a weekly plan. I do this every Sunday: I look at the week I've got coming up and plan to fit in my workouts accordingly. So, for example, if you're going out with your mate on Wednesday night and you usually do your workouts then, schedule a morning workout that day.

I like writing my workout schedule down in an old-school planner, but it's totally up to you how you do it. Whether it's on your phone, on a whiteboard, on a piece of paper you stick on your fridge – whatever! Just make sure you write out your workout plan each week. You're then much more likely to commit and stick to it.

3. Set your goals

Goals are massively important because they give you something to work towards. They give you a desired result you can visualise, a target to reach, and this will keep you motivated to keep on with your exercise programme, especially if you're going through a tricky phase where you just want to quit.

You've got to make your goals realistic, though, so they can motivate you properly. In the same way that you'd never make a ridiculous goal like 'I wanna earn a million pounds in a month', you should never make an exercise goal like 'I wanna lose 3 stone in a month by exercising with Courtney'. That's not gonna happen! If you set unrealistic goals, you'll end up disappointed and give up. You're going to have to change it up. Look at what a realistic goal would be. That way, you'll make a meaningful change that will last for life.

Short- and long-term goals

I recommend giving yourself a mixture of short-term goals and long-term goals. Short-term goals are the ones that keep you on track because they're achievable in quicker times, so they keep you motivated. Good examples of short-term goals could be:

By the end of the week I want to:

☑ be able to run for ten minutes without stopping

☑ have done all the workouts

☑ feel 10 per cent fitter in myself

They don't even have to be this big! A great short-term goal could be 'I want to do a whole workout today and not give up halfway through'. The point is, they are ways that you can see the results of your efforts in a quicker timeframe.

Long-term goals are the ones that take time to achieve – you don't hit them as easily. They're the gold medals at the end of the marathon. Some examples of long-term goals could be:

☑ I want to fit into my wedding dress

☑ I want to do an Iron Man Triathlon

☑ I want to improve my resting heart rate from X to X

☑ I want to run a marathon

☑ I want to reduce my cholesterol from X to X

☑ I want to reverse my type 2 diabetes

You've got to mix them up. If you just have long-term goals, you can lose your way, as they can feel impossible to achieve, especially in the early days; if you just have short-term goals, you can lose momentum if you've achieved them too easily.

Hitting your goals – both short- and long-term – gives you an amazing sense of achievement. Maybe give yourself a treat if you hit your goal, something like buying yourself a nice top, or a trip to the cinema. Whatever it is, make it something you'll really enjoy, something that will remind you that you've earned this!

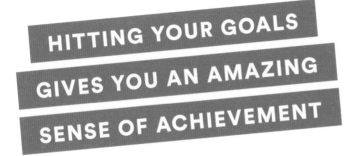

HITTING YOUR GOALS GIVES YOU AN AMAZING SENSE OF ACHIEVEMENT

Use SMART planning

Deciding on your goals can be a tricky one. To make sure I come up with ones that will work for me, I always use SMART goal planning. It's an acronym tool that you can use to plan out relevant goals – making sure that it hits each of the SMART criteria. They are:

S – SPECIFIC
M – MEASURABLE
A – ACHIEVABLE
R – RELEVANT
T – TIME-BOUND

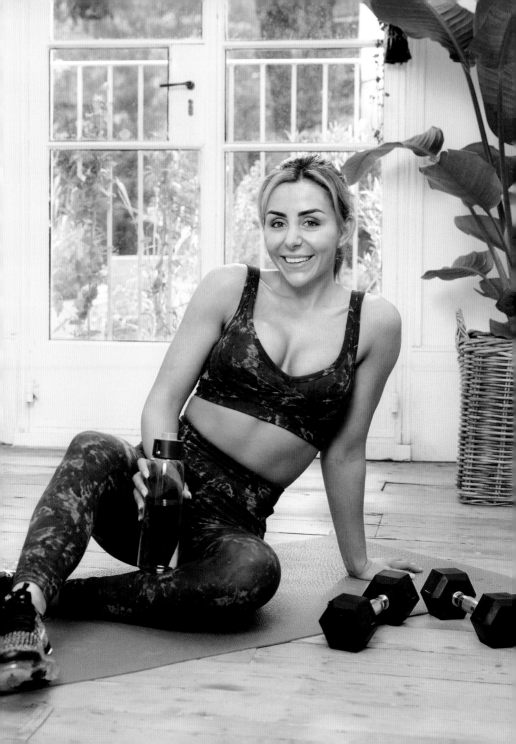

Okay, so here's an example of a SMART goal to help you see how they work. Imagine you're a total beginner to exercise. Your SMART goal could be 'I want to complete three hours of Courtney workouts in one week'. This is a really great goal because:

It's specific – the goal is focused on one particular type of exercise.

It's measurable – the three hours of time means that you can easily see if you're hitting it.

It's achievable – three hours in a week is really doable. Thirty hours? Not so much!

It's relevant – you're setting fitness-based goals, and this is an ideal one.

It's time-bound – you've given yourself a deadline, which gives you something concrete to work towards.

But make them goals for YOU!

A mistake I used to make in my younger days was that my goals were all about other people. So, for example, when I was working in an office job, my goal was to earn enough money to buy certain things to impress other people. Or when I was dealing with my eating disorder, my goal was to look a certain way to impress a boy. It was crazy, but that was the way my brain was wired back then.

The problem with making your goals all about other people is that you don't stick to them, and their success is down to the behaviour of others. So, for example, if you're trying to impress a guy and he goes, your goal has gone; if you're trying to be as skinny as your mate, and you fall out, well ... what then?

Make sure your goals are about you, your aims and achievements. They're things you can do for you, to make you feel better, and not because you're trying to be someone else. You're trying to be the best version of yourself. So set your goals, and fight for them.

Get a good night's rest

You might be thinking to yourself, what on earth has sleeping got to do with exercise, Court? But I'm here to tell you it's got everything to do with it! Sleep affects every part of your life – your stress, your mindset, your energy levels. It gives your body time to recover and repair after you've exercised, so it's vital to get a decent amount of sleep every night.

There has been so much research done into the effects that poor sleep can have on your mind and body, so if you want to achieve your fitness goals, you've got to make sure you're getting enough sleep. Aim for at least seven hours each night – if not more – and make sure you get into a regular cycle of going to bed and getting up at similar times each day.

Understanding your natural sleep cycle will also be really helpful in working out when you should exercise. If you're a lark like me, then it's obvious you should work out in the morning – but if you're the type of night owl who can't turn out the light until 1am, then don't set your alarm for a 6am workout! On the other hand, if you've had a rough night's sleep, don't give up on that day's exercise, just get through it and you'll probably find you sleep even better that following night – because you're properly tired!

Affirmations

I love affirmations! Simply put, they're positive statements that reinforce self-worth. They make you believe that there is a place in the world for you. By putting positive affirmations out into the world, it's the first step in making them actually happen, because you begin to believe them yourself.

I first came across affirmations when I was working in the City. All the boys there loved them – that's how I discovered the book by Brian Tracy and also a really famous book called *The Secret* by Rhonda Byrne. Reading these opened my mind to using affirmations positively – by changing my thoughts about myself, I could change my behaviour.

Affirmations should be personal to you, and they can be used for anything, not just exercise. But here are some examples so you can see what I mean:

— I am successful
— I am determined
— I am physically fit
— I am healthy
— I am going to smash this workout

Do you see how they can help? Instead of saying something negative to yourself like, 'Oh, I'm dreading this workout, it's going to be awful,' you make it a positive thing. I believe they give you the right approach and set you up to succeed far more than a negative mindset.

If you say them over and over again, they soon become a habit. These days I don't consciously wake up in the morning and start saying my affirmations; they've just become part of my life, and are part of the reason that I'm such a positive person now.

So start thinking about your own affirmations. What would motivate you? What could you tell yourself to make you feel better? Write them down, start telling them to yourself, repeat them in your head – whatever it is that will help you start internalising this really positive message. Affirmations are truly individual, and what works for me might not work for you, so spend a little time coming up with the brilliantly positive affirmations that are gonna help you focus on achieving your fitness goals.

AFFIRMATIONS SET YOU UP TO SUCCEED

PART FOUR – YOUR 28-DAY FITNESS PLAN

Hey, team! You're now ready to start on your fitness journey with me and become the healthiest, happiest and fittest version of you. That's an amazing, amazing thing to have decided upon in the first place, so you can feel good about that right away!

Okay, a few things before we kick off ...

Tracking your progress

It's really important to be able to chart the progress you make during the 28 days you'll be following the plan. I'm not a fan of scales – they're misleading in terms of fitness because they only show weight lost or gained. If you see the scales go up a bit, it's gonna make you feel really demotivated, but in fact, you might have got loads fitter – so, chuck out the scales and instead try these other ways to monitor how you're going to get fitter and stronger:

- **Take photos:** Before, during and after photos are an easy and encouraging way to see how your body changes. Take photos of yourself from front and side-on (and the back, if you have someone who can do it for you!). Re-take them each week from the same angles throughout the plan. Resist the temptation to filter them; the whole point of this is to honestly track your progress. You don't have to put this up online either if you don't want to – it's totally up to you. But if you find it motivating to post it on your Insta, tag me and go for it!

- **Measure yourself:** Grab a tape measure and see how you measure up round key parts of your body, and track this in a chart. Again, only do this once a week and do it at the same time each week. Our bodies are changeable so be consistent in terms of when you measure. You should write down measurements for your:

  — **Waist – around the belly button**
  — **Hips – choose the widest part around your bum**
  — **Thigh – just choose left or right but make sure you measure the same one each week!**
  — **Upper arm – same as above**

- **Chart your achievements:** You're gonna find working out harder to start with, that's natural. A great way not to feel down about it is to chart how much you improve over time. So if you can only do two push-ups in a row to begin with, don't worry, write it down. If you can only do five squat jumps without needing to take a break, write that down. If you can only run for 30 seconds without tiring, write it down! Then track those exercises week by week to see how many more you can do as you get fitter. The numbers will go up, I promise. It's so motivating to see how much longer you can go on and how many more reps you can do!

I'VE NOTICED SUCH A MASSIVE POSITIVE CHANGE IN MY BODY

Body language

There are a few terms I use when you work out. In case you don't know what they are, here's a quick glossary!

Abs	Your front stomach muscles
Biceps	Your front upper-arm muscles
Lats	Your back and shoulders area
Obliques	Your side stomach muscles
Triceps	Your back upper-arm muscles (bingo wings!)
Glutes	Your bum, basically!
Reps	Short for 'repetitions', it's the number of times you do a single exercise without stopping for a rest

Why HIIT and weights?

You'll notice that most of the workout sessions are a combination of HIIT (high-intensity interval training) circuits, plus some weight training at the end in the 'finisher' section. So why do I recommend this type of training? Actually, I never used to do HIIT sessions much before I started the home workouts in lockdown, but I've noticed such a massive, positive change in my body, it's crazy. The reason they're good is that they're quick, short and effective, and focus on bursts of hard work.

You don't have to spend that long doing the workouts – each one averages out at around 30 minutes, and that's enough – but during that time you can bust such a sweat, burn loads of calories and shape your body so amazingly! You'll hit your legs, your arms and your core in movements that target these areas and improve overall fitness.

Another reason HIIT workouts are so effective is because they cause the EPOC effect. This is a technical term that stands for 'excess post-exercise oxygen consumption'. It means that doing these exercises raises your resting metabolic rate, so that you're burning more calories even after you've trained. Amazing, isn't it? As well as this, when you pair the weight training with it – the finisher sections – you're building muscle mass. The more muscle you have, the more efficient your body becomes at burning energy at rest, too. I also like to split out the muscle groups in the workouts, because this is more effective at sculpting your body than just doing pure cardio. I love these combinations of exercises and they are absolutely brilliant for you.

☑ CHECK IN ON YOUR HEALTH

If you have any health issues or concerns, please check with your GP before starting the exercise plan. You don't want to do anything that will make you ill or damage your body. Take care of yourself!

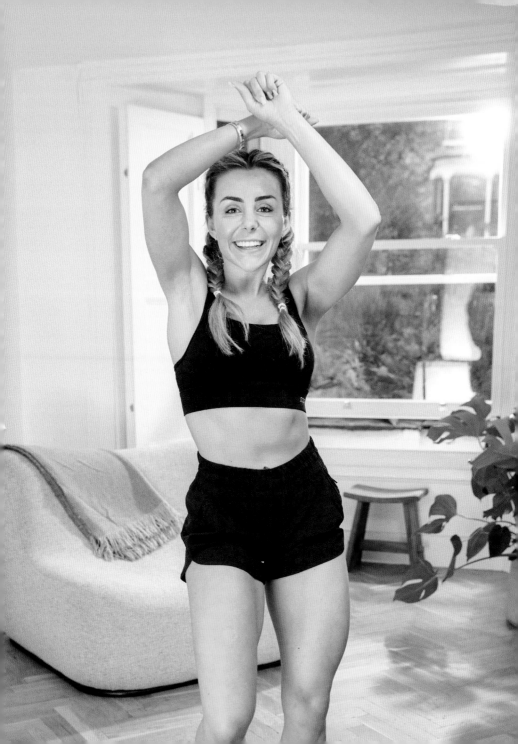

WARMING UP + COOLING DOWN

Before every single workout you should always do a five-minute warm-up, and then a few minutes cool-down at the end. Warming up and cooling down is so important as it raises then reduces your body temperature and increases blood flow to your muscles. It will also reduce recovery time and reduce muscle soreness. There's a difference, though, between the types of warming-up and cooling-down exercises you should do in each section. When warming up you never want to do static stretches (as you would when cooling down) – you want to get your heart rate up and your body moving! Whereas with cool-downs, you need to stretch out every muscle you've been working during the session.

MY EASY WARM-UP

These active exercises are perfect to get you ready to start my workouts. Do them all, but you can mix up the order however you want.

30-SECOND JOG ON THE SPOT

Imagine that you are on a treadmill or on the ground travelling, and jog exactly as you would, but without moving forwards. Pick your feet up and get a good pace going.

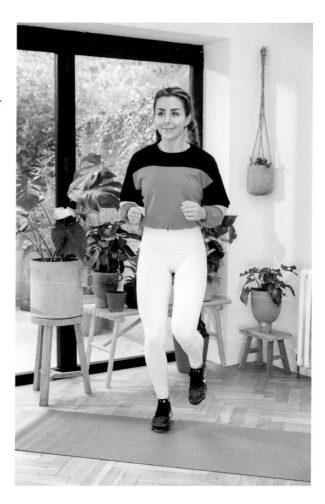

MY EASY WARM-UP
10 SQUATS

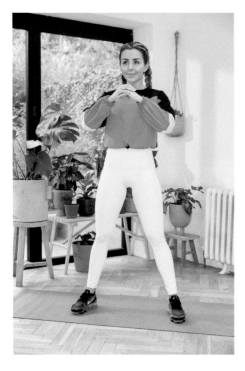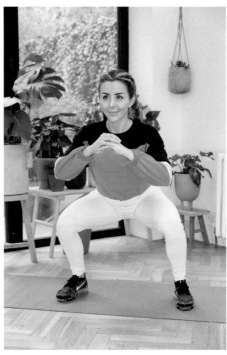

Start in standing position with your feet wider than shoulder-width, chest up, hands clasped in front of you and your core engaged. Squat down until your knees are parallel with your hips, keeping your knees in line and not dropping your chest. Return to standing position, pushing your weight through your heels. Repeat ten times.

30-SECOND JOG

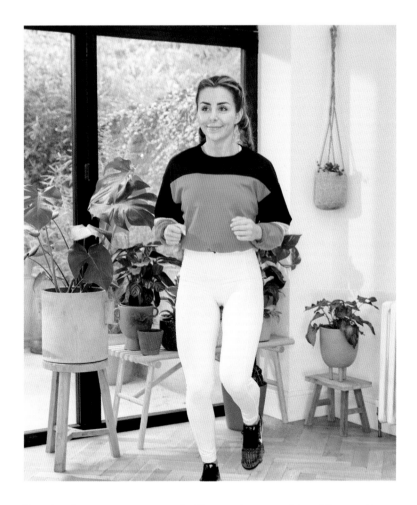

Imagine that you are on a treadmill or on the ground travelling, and jog exactly as you would, but without moving forwards. Pick your feet up and get a good pace going.

10 STAR JUMPS

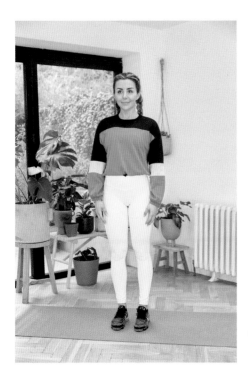
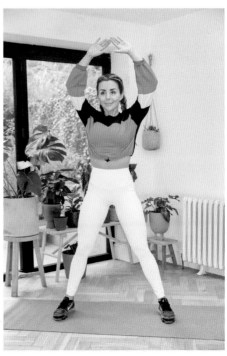

Start in standing position with your feet together and arms by your side. Jump your feet out to slightly further apart than your shoulders and simultaneously raise your arms above your head. Return to standing position, with feet together, and repeat for a total of ten reps.

5 LUNGES
WITH A HIGH-REACH STRETCH PER SIDE

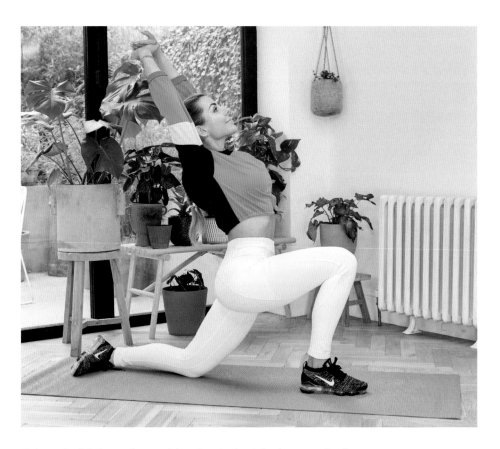

Take a nice big lunge forward, leaving the back leg knee on the floor. Drive your hip forward into the front leg and reach up with your arms above your head for a big, deep stretch. Repeat on the other leg, for a total of 5 times each side.

10 SHOULDER ROLLS

BACKWARDS AND FORWARDS

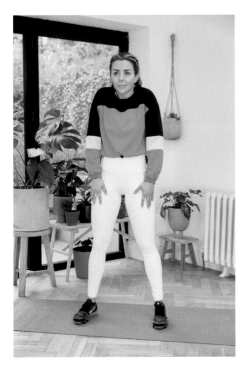 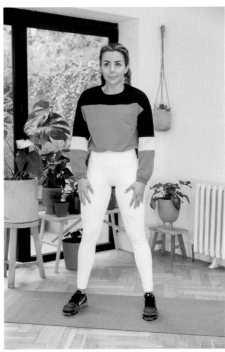

Place your arms down by your side and, keeping them straight as possible, roll your arms forwards and backwards in big circular motions. Do it ten times in either direction.

THE IDEAL COOL-DOWN

These stretches are my favourite for stretching every muscle, and will take no more than five minutes. Spend 30–60 seconds on each stretch.

KNEELING HIP FLEXOR STRETCH

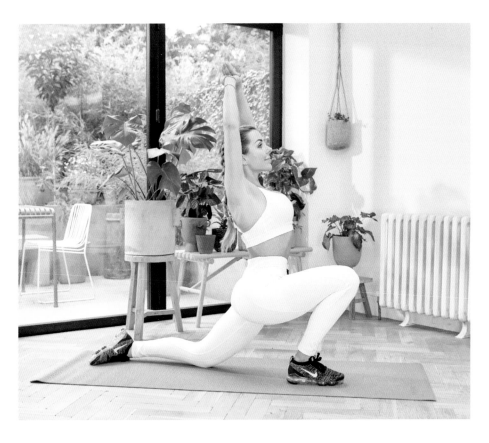

Put your right leg forward, foot on the floor, and left leg back with your left knee on the floor, creating a 90-degree angle with both legs bent at the knee. Push your hips forward, keep your chest upright, tuck your hips under and push both arms up into a high stretch. Lower your arms, swap the position of the legs and repeat.

PECTORAL WALL STRETCH

Put one hand on a wall, a door or anything sturdy, arm straight, and stretch out your chest. Your body should be facing away from your hand. Really rotate your torso and feel the stretch. Swap hands and stretch in the other direction.

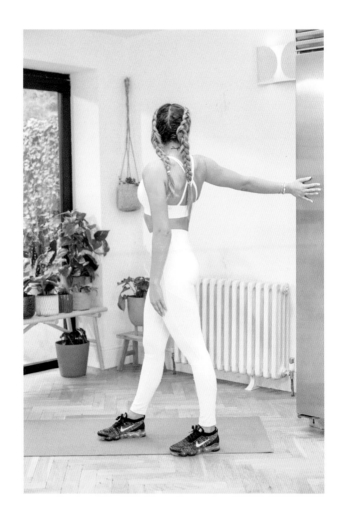

LYING FIGURE-4 STRETCH

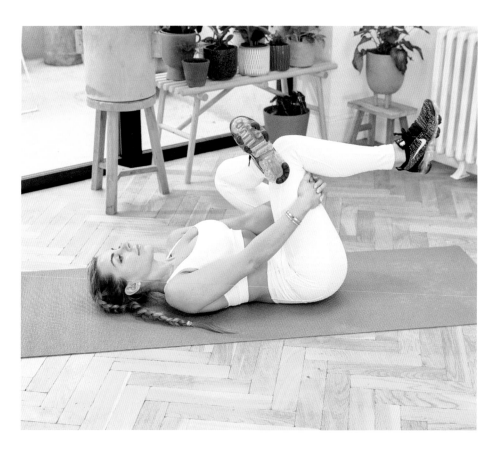

Lying on your mat, cross your left foot over your right knee, bring your right leg up to a 90-degree angle and joining your hands under your right leg, clasping them around your hamstring. Keep your left knee open away from your body to feel a deep glute stretch. Return the legs to the floor and repeat with your other leg.

THE IDEAL COOL-DOWN
SHOULDER CROSS STRETCH

Put your right arm across your chest and lock it in with your left arm on your right arm, just above the elbow. Keep your head straight and shoulders down. Repeat with your right arm.

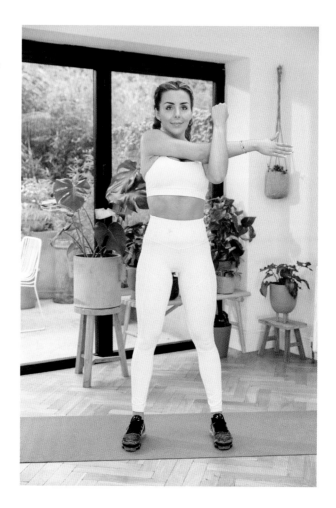

THE IDEAL COOL-DOWN
STANDING CALF STRETCH

Stand near a wall or sturdy surface with one foot directly in front and in line with the other, front knee slightly bent. Keep your back leg straight. Put your hands on the wall or surface, at shoulder level, keeping your chest up, then lean towards your hands. Return to standing, swap legs and repeat.

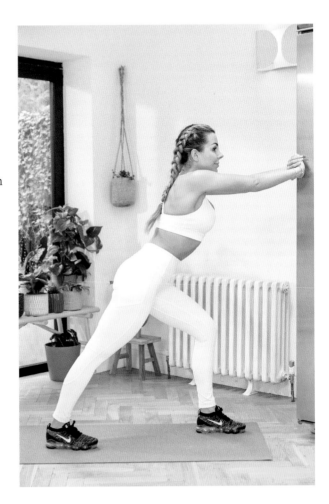

THE IDEAL COOL-DOWN
OVERHEAD TRICEPS STRETCH

Reach your right arm up to the ceiling, bend your elbow to bring your hand down your back. With your left hand pull your right elbow to stretch your tricep. Repeat on the other side.

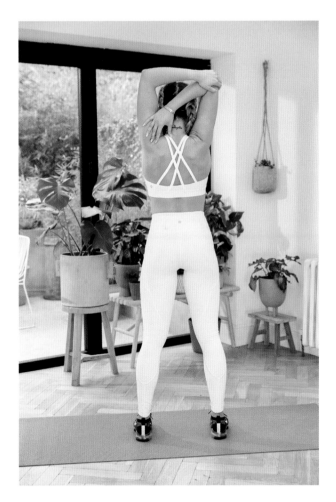

THE IDEAL COOL-DOWN
QUAD STRETCH

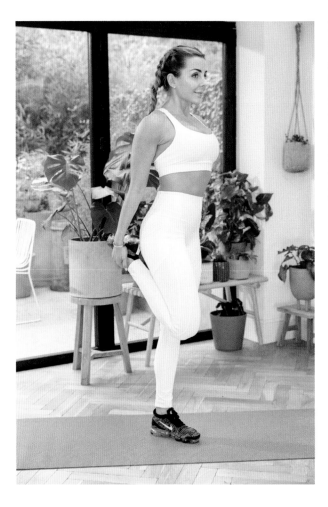

Hold your outside foot with your outside hand and lift it up to your butt, keeping your knees together (place your other hand on a wall for balance if you need to). Return your foot to the floor and repeat the stretch with the other hand and leg.

THE IDEAL COOL-DOWN
HAMSTRING/CALF STRETCH

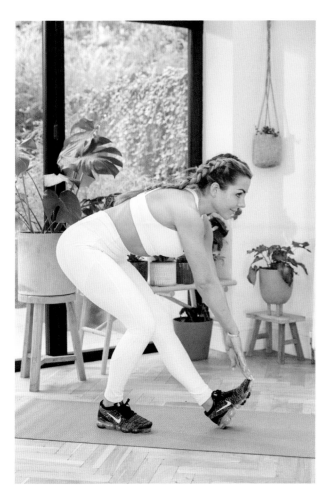

Place your left foot directly in front of you and push your hips back to lean your torso forward, extending the right leg. Flex your left ankle so your toes are pointing upwards and touch your toes with your fingertips. Repeat with the other leg.

EXERCISE GUIDE

Before you start the plan, here are explanations and pictures of all the exercises I'm going to include in the workouts.

AB EXERCISES

RUSSIAN TWISTS

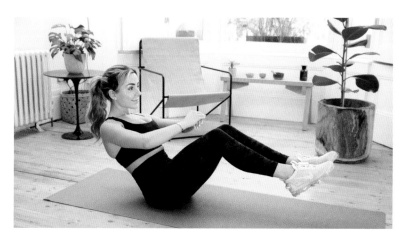

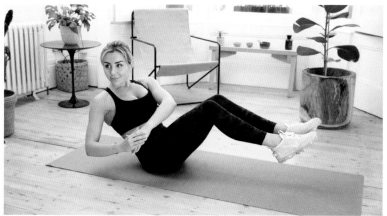

Sit on the floor, bend your legs and lift your legs off the ground. Rotate your torso, reaching your left elbow towards your right knee. Repeat on the other side.

CRUNCHES

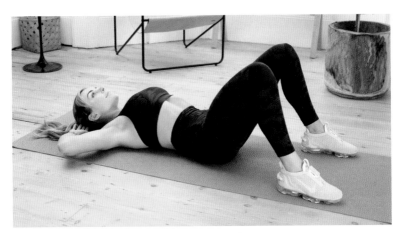

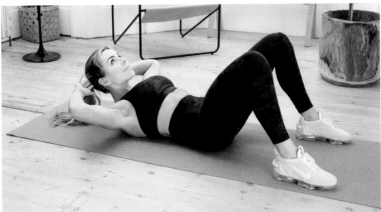

Lie on your back on your mat, hands on either side of your head near your temples and keep your arms in this position (elbows to the side). Keep your eyes and your head up at all times, avoiding putting chin to chest. Engage your core so your shoulders come up off the floor. Hold at the top of the contraction for two seconds before slowly lowering.

SIT-UPS

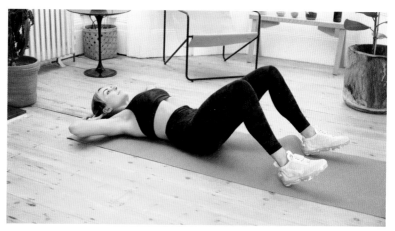

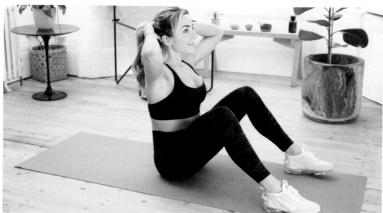

Lie on your back with your legs bent, your feet flat on the floor hip-width apart, and your back pressed flat against your mat. Place your hands either side of your head or across your shoulders, then curl your torso up to your knees, but avoid straining your neck. Slowly lower back down, keeping your core engaged.

LEG RAISES

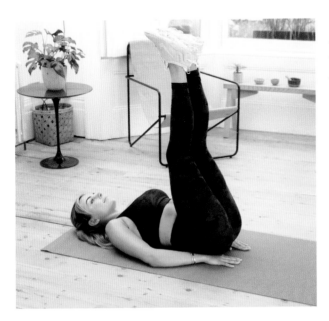

Lie on your back with your legs straight and your back pressed flat against your mat. Keep your legs as straight as possible and lift them all the way up to the ceiling until your butt comes off the floor. Slowly lower your legs down but do not let them touch the floor. Repeat.

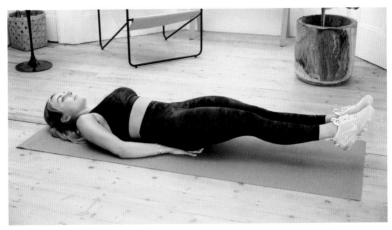

PLANK HIP ROTATIONS

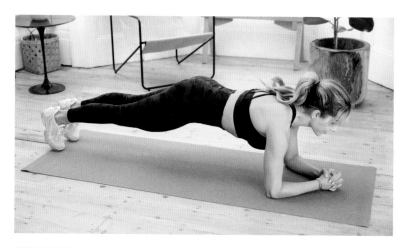

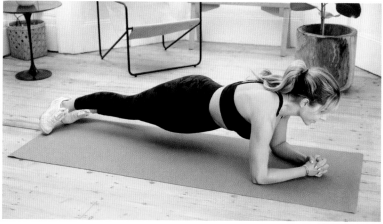

Start on your forearms in a low plank position. Pull in your abs as you rotate your hips to the left and tap the floor with your hips, then rotate to the right and tap the floor on the other side.

BICYCLE CRUNCHES

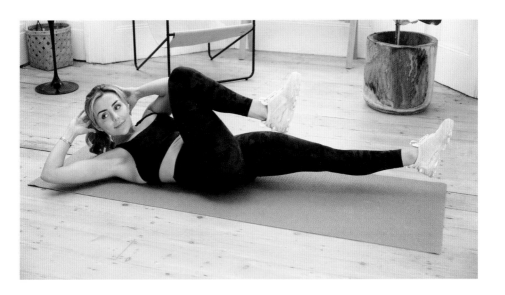

Lie on your back on your mat. Press your lower back against your mat and place your hands on your head, elbows to the side. Bring your knees into your chest and lift your shoulders off the ground. Straighten your left leg, elevating it slightly, while rotating your torso and bringing your left elbow to your right knee (keeping your hands on your head). Switch sides.

SIT-UP RUSSIAN TWISTS

Lie on your back with your legs bent and your back pressed flat against your mat. Place your hands either side of your head or clasp them across your torso. Curl your torso up to your knees, legs bent, and twist your torso left and right before slowly lowering back down, keeping your core engaged. Repeat.

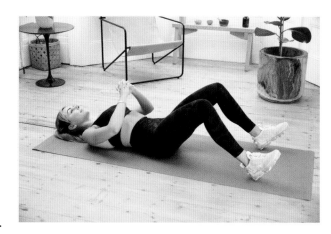

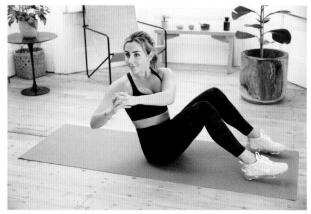

TUCKS

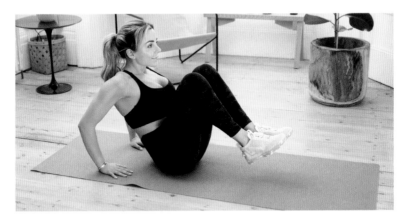

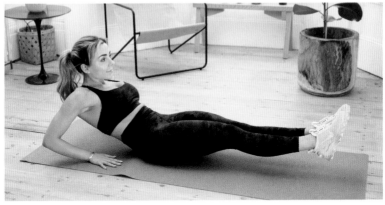

Sit so your legs are bent, feet on the floor, and you are leaning halfway back with your hands on the mat behind you. Extend your legs out straight, keeping them off the floor slightly. On each rep tuck your legs into your stomach and come forward with your torso. Extend back out and repeat.

V-UPS

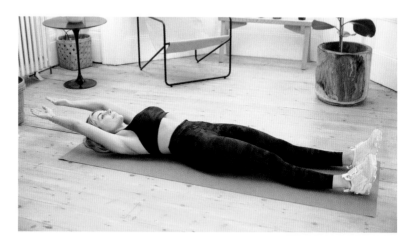

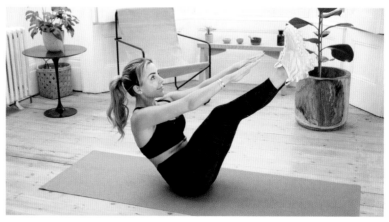

Lie on your back on your mat with your legs and arms straight, holding your arms above your head and keeping your feet on the floor. In one movement lift your torso and legs together, trying to touch your toes to create a 'V' shape. Lower back down and repeat.

COMMANDOS

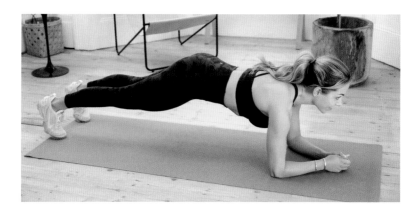

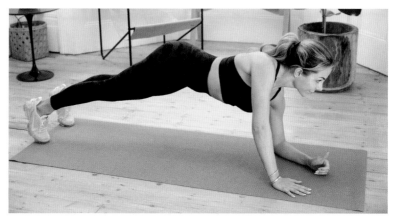

Start on your forearms in a low plank position. Lift your right forearm to place your hand firmly on the mat directly below your right shoulder and push up onto your right hand. Lift your left forearm, too, so you're now in a high plank. Release your right hand and lower your forearm to the mat, then release your left hand and lower your forearm to the mat to return to the starting position. Repeat.

LEG EXERCISES

BODYWEIGHT SQUATS

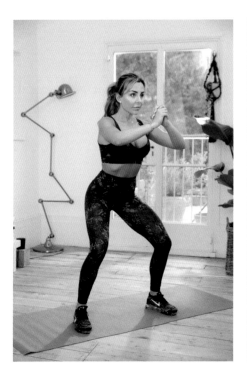
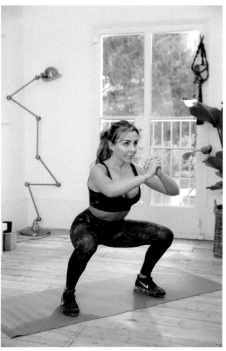

Start in standing position with your feet wider than shoulder-width, chest up, hands clasped in front of you and your core engaged. Squat down until your knees are parallel with your hips, keeping your knees in line and not dropping your chest. Return to standing position, pushing your weight through your heels. Repeat.

DUMBBELL REVERSE LUNGES

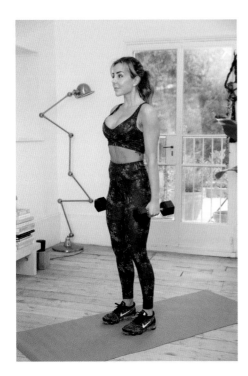
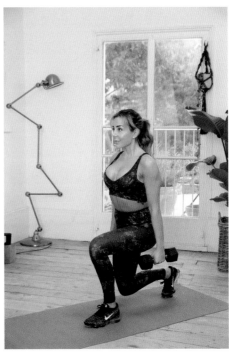

Start in standing position, holding a dumbbell in each hand, palms facing your body, with your feet hip-width apart and arms by your side. Take a large step backwards, lowering your back knee towards the ground and keeping your core engaged and chest up. Bring yourself back to standing position by pushing through your front heel and repeat with the other leg.

CURTSY LUNGES WITH DUMBBELL BICEP CURLS

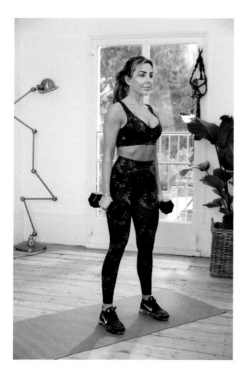
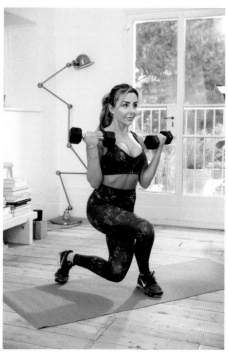

Start in standing position, holding a dumbbell in each hand by your side, with your palms facing your body, chest up and feet hip-width apart. Shift your weight onto your stationary foot, then step the other leg back and to the side, behind your stationary leg, in a diagonal movement. Bend both knees as you lunge and curl your biceps up. Push through your heel on the back foot to return to standing. Repeat, switching legs each time you lunge.

STRAIGHT-LEG DEADLIFTS WITH DUMBBELLS

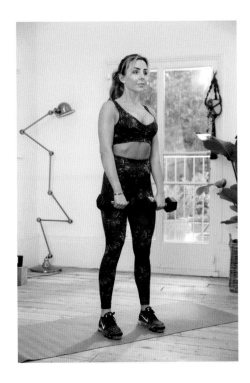
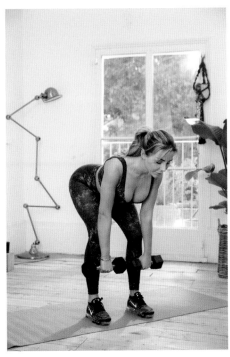

Start in standing position, holding a dumbbell in each hand with your palms facing your body, chest up and feet hip-width apart. Lower the dumbbells by bending at the waist and pushing your hips back, with straight legs but knees soft. Return upright by lifting your chest and pushing through your glutes and heels. Repeat.

POWER SQUATS

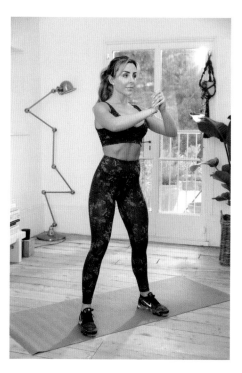 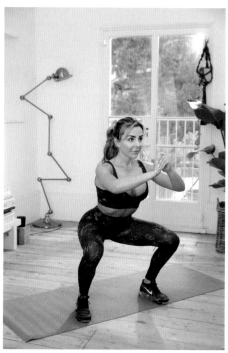

Start in standing position with your feet wide and hands clasped in front of you. Squat down and touch the floor with your fingertips, then jump up as high as you can and take your arms up above your head as you do so. Repeat.

GOBLET SQUATS WITH DUMBELLS

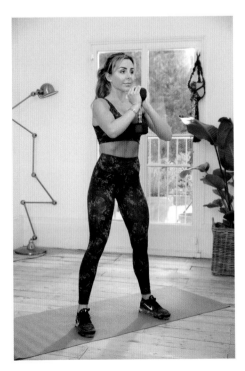
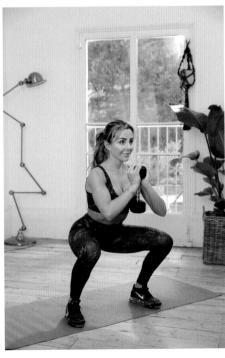

Hold a dumbbell or two dumbbells to your chest. Position your feet so the stance is wider than shoulder-width and turn your toes out a little. Squat down until your hips and knees are parallel, making sure you keep your chest up. As you stand, push through your heels and squeeze your butt at the top. Repeat.

DUMBBELL GLUTE BRIDGES

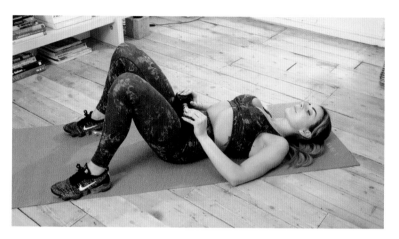

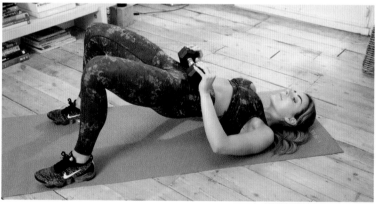

Lie on your back on your mat, knees bent and feet on the floor, and hold a dumbbell in each hand, or one dumbbell, resting the dumbbell(s) above your hip bones. Squeeze your glutes and abs and push through your heels to lift your hips off the floor until your body forms a straight diagonal line from your shoulders to your knees. Squeeze your glutes and hold for a few seconds before slowly lowering. Repeat.

SPLIT SQUATS WITH DUMBBELLS

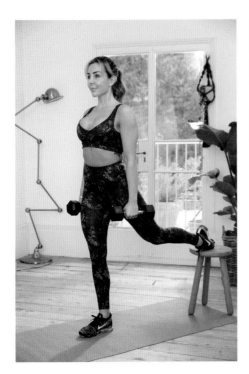 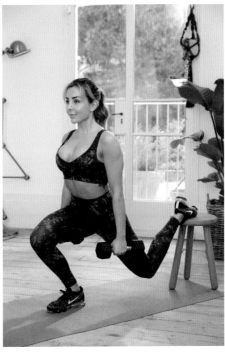

Start in standing position, in front of a stool, chair or sofa, with a dumbbell in each hand. Lift one leg behind you so the top of your foot is resting on the stool, chair or sofa. Take a wider stance for better glute activation. Bend the front knee as low as you can, then push through your heel to return to an upright position and squeeze your glutes at the top. Repeat.

REVERSE DUMBBELL LUNGES WITH PULSES

Start in standing position, holding a dumbbell in each hand by your side, with your palms facing your body and your feet hip-width apart. Take a large step backwards, lowering your back knee towards the ground and keeping your core engaged and chest up. Pulse halfway up before lowering back down. Bring yourself back to standing by pushing through your front heel and repeat with the other leg.

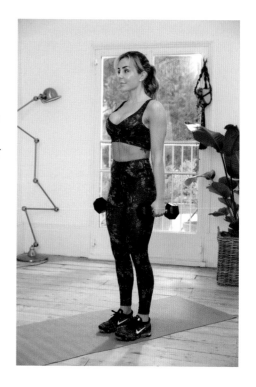

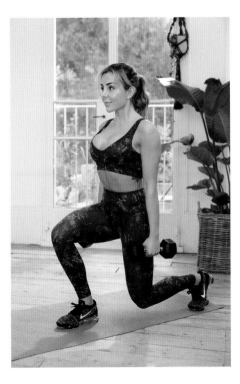
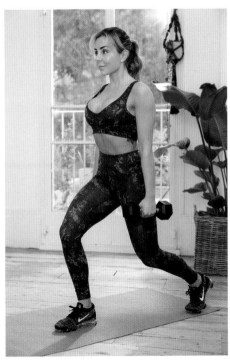

CURTSY LUNGES WITH DUMBBELLS

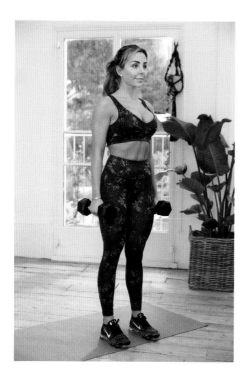
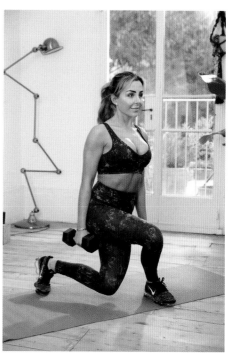

Start in standing position, holding a dumbbell in each hand by your side, with your palms facing your body and your feet hip-width apart. Shift your weight onto your stationary foot, then step the other leg back and to the side, behind your stationary leg, in a diagonal movement. Bend both knees as you lunge down. Push through your heel on the back foot to return to standing. Repeat, switching legs each time you lunge.

LATERAL LUNGES

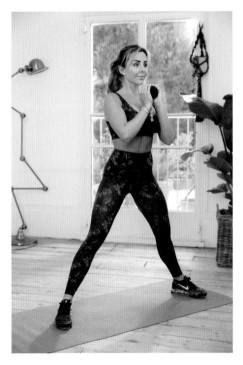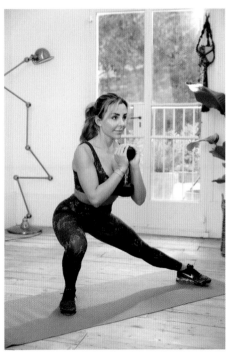

Hold a dumbbell and take a wide leg position. Lunge into one leg, staying low, then swing to the other leg and repeat.

REVERSE LUNGE WITH KNEE DRIVES

Start in standing position with your feet hip-width apart, arms held in front of your chest, and step your left foot back, coming into a reverse lunge. Shift all of your weight to your right foot, engaging your glutes. Bring your left foot forward and simultaneously jump off your right foot, bringing your left knee into your chest. Step back into a lunge and repeat.

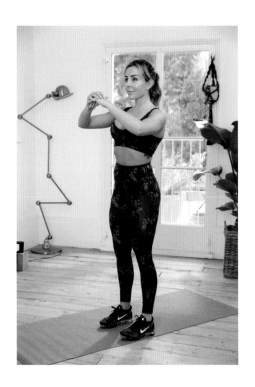

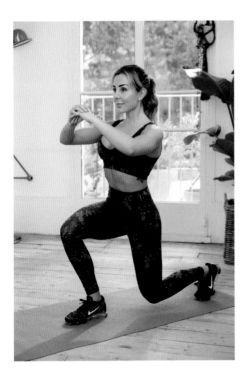
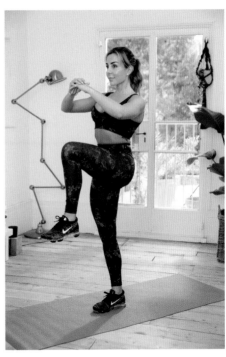

ARM EXERCISES

BODYWEIGHT RENEGADE ROWS

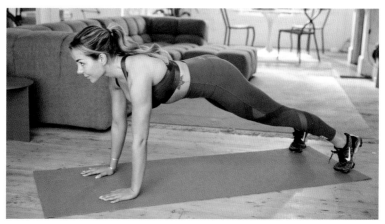

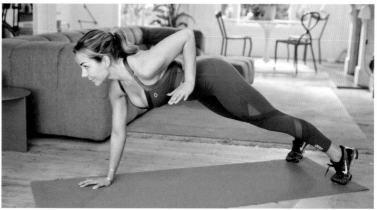

Start in a high plank position with hands placed on the floor directly under the shoulders and feet shoulder-width apart. Keep one hand pushing firmly into the floor as you pull the other up to your waist (bending at the elbow and squeezing your lats). Lower your arm to the floor and repeat with the opposite arm.

BICEP CURLS INTO SHOULDER PRESSES WITH DUMBBELLS

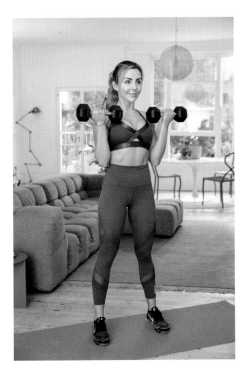 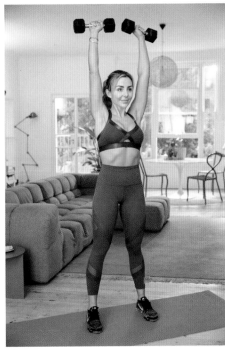

Start in standing position, holding a dumbbell in each hand, and curl your arms up to your shoulders, using your biceps, keeping your elbows by your side. Twist your palms out so you can get into a starting shoulder-press position and push your arms up. Lower the dumbbells with control and repeat.

LATERAL RAISES WITH DUMBBELLS

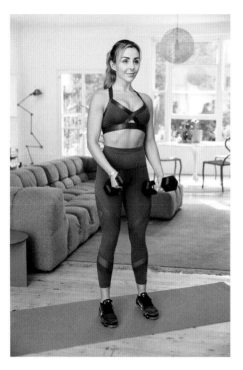 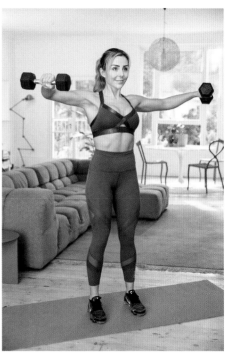

Start in standing position with a dumbbell in each hand. Raise the dumbbells upwards, away from your body (slightly bending at the elbows), with your palms facing the floor. Lower the dumbbells with control, then repeat.

LYING CHEST PRESS WITH DUMBBELLS

Lie on your back on your mat with a dumbbell in each hand and knees bent. Start with the dumbbells at shoulder width and level, with your palms facing away from you. Use your chest and arms to push the dumbbells up, locking your elbows at the top of the movement. Lower the weight slowly and in a controlled way. Repeat.

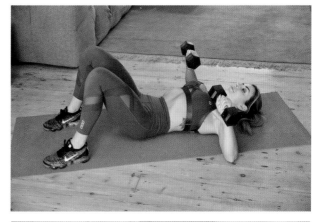

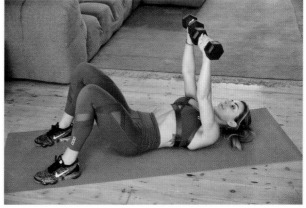

DUMBBELL UPRIGHT ROW

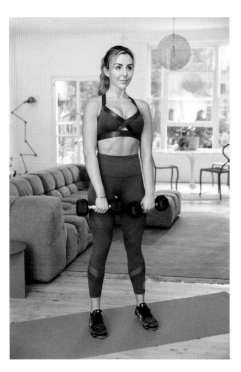
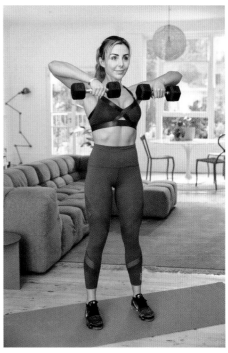

Start in standing position with a dumbbell in each hand, with your palms facing your body. Use your shoulders to raise the dumbbells up to shoulder/chest level (elbows up), while bending your arms. Lower the dumbbells back down and repeat.

ARM EXERCISES
DUMBBELL FLYES

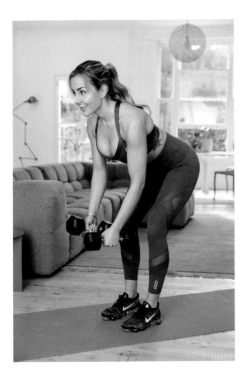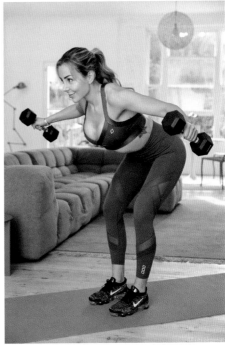

Start in standing position with a dumbbell in each hand, and hinge your chest forward from the hips so your back is flat, and you have a slight bend in your knees. You can also do this sitting on the edge of a chair if it is easier for you. Let the dumbbells hang straight down from your shoulders, keeping your palms facing one another. Raise your arms straight (with a slight bend at the elbow) out to the side, pinching your back muscles (lats) together. Lower the dumbbells with control and repeat.

BENT-OVER ROWS WITH DUMBBELLS

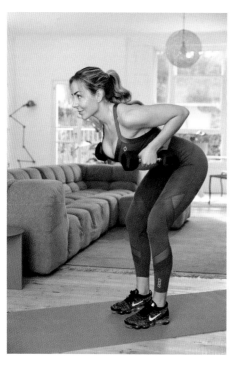
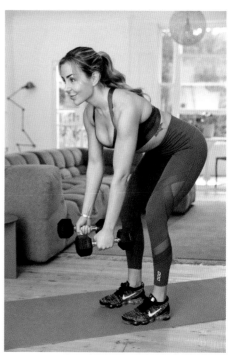

Start in standing position with a dumbbell in each hand, palms facing your body. The dumbbells should be held shoulder-width apart, in parallel with your feet. Bend your knees slightly and hinge your chest forward from the hips so your back is flat. Pull the dumbbells up to your stomach by tucking your elbows in and squeezing your lats. Lower the dumbbells with control and repeat.

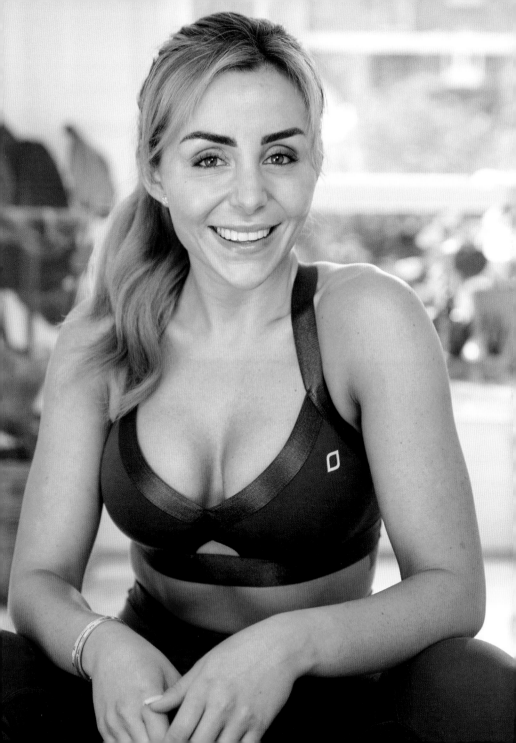

ARM EXERCISES
PRESS-UPS

Start in a standard press-up position. Place your hands on the floor slightly wider than shoulder-width apart. Slowly lower your chest towards the floor while ensuring your abs are tight. Push back up to return to start position. If you find press-ups really hard, then you can do them on your knees: start in a table position, with your ankles crossed over, then lean down and lower your chest towards the floor as above.

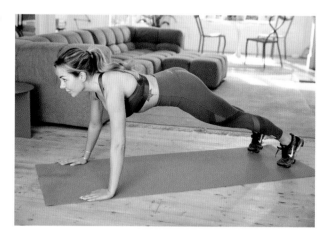

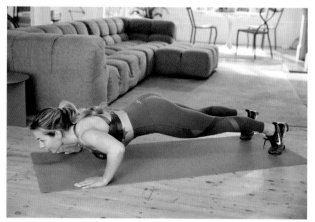

RENEGADE ROW WITH DUMBBELLS

Start in a high plank position with each hand grasping a dumbbell on the floor. Keep one hand pushing firmly into the dumbbell as you pull the other up to your waist (bending at the elbow and squeezing your lats). Lower your arm to the floor and repeat with the opposite arm.

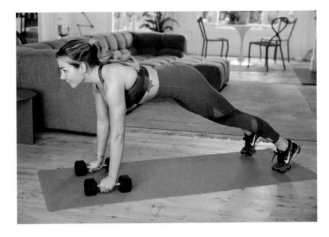

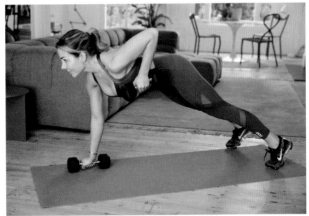

SHOULDER PRESS

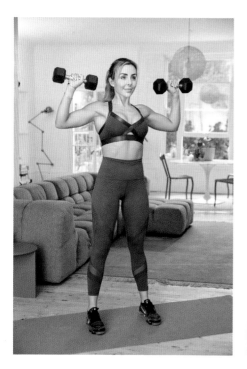 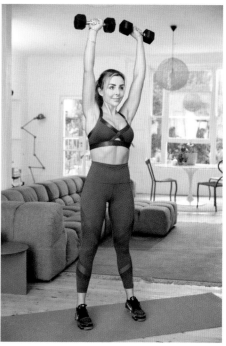

Start in standing position holding a dumbbell in each hand at shoulder level, with your palms facing away from you. Press the weights up, then slowly lower them back down. Aim to press the weights above your head rather than out to the side.

CLOSE-GRIP DUMBBELL PRESSES

Lie on your mat, with your knees bent, and hold a dumbbell in each hand above your chest, with your arms straight but elbows not locked, and your palms facing each other. Slowly lower the weights down to your chest, keeping your elbows tucked in, then press back up.

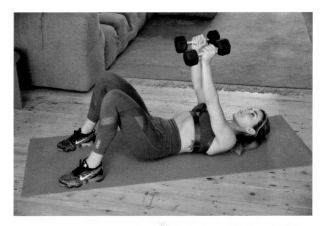

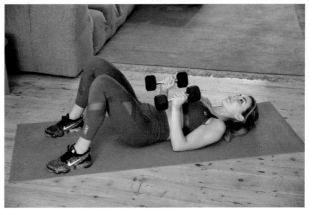

CARDIO EXERCISES

REVERSE-LUNGE LEG DRIVES

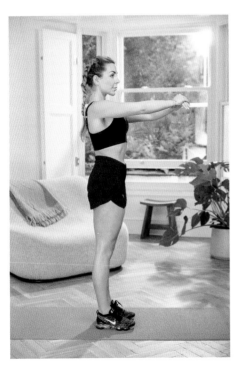
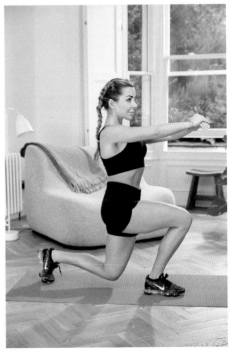

Start in standing position with your feet hip-width apart, arms held in front of your chest, and step your left foot back, coming into a reverse lunge. Shift all of your weight to your right foot, engaging your glutes. Bring your left foot forward and simultaneously jump off your right foot, bringing your left knee up to your chest. Step back into a lunge with the other leg and repeat.

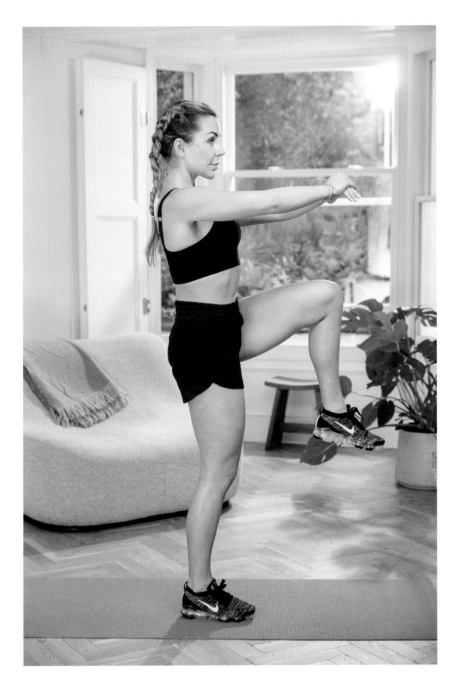

CARDIO EXERCISES
JUMP LUNGES

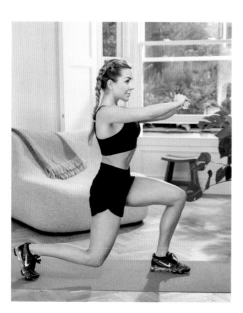
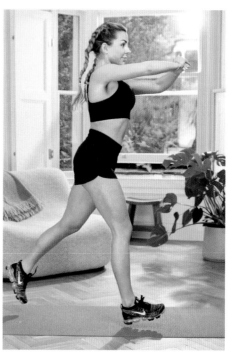

Start in standing position with one leg forward and one leg back. Hold your arms in front of your chest with your elbows bent ready. Prepare to jump by bending your knees and lunging down (slightly leaning forward will improve balance and core contraction). Explosively launch your body up, extending your knees and hips to straighten your legs as you change legs, then lower back down into a lunge on the opposite leg. Repeat, alternating legs.

SQUAT JACKS

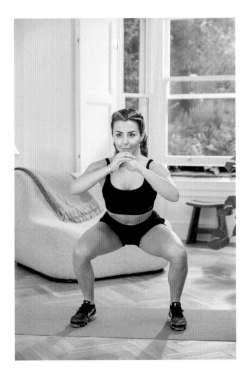 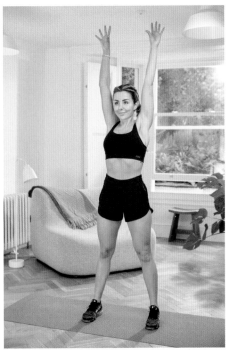

Start in standing position with your feet together, then jump down into a wide squat and touch your ankles. As you jump back up to standing, raise your arms above your head. Repeat.

SQUAT JUMPS

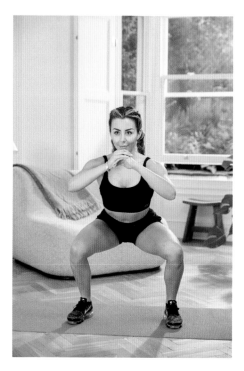
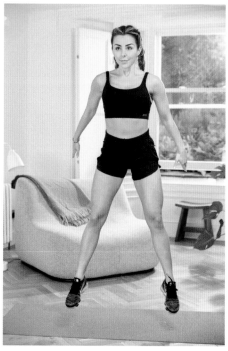

Start in standing position with your feet wide, and bend into a squat position. Jump into the air and land back in the squat position. Make sure you do not let your knees cave in towards each other – keep them facing forward. Push through your heels to return to standing position and repeat.

SQUAT THRUSTERS

Start in a high plank position, then jump your feet into a wide squat and bring your hands off the ground and to your chest. Pause for a second, replace hands to the ground and jump back into your high plank. If you find the jumping part really hard, you can step forward with your feet instead. Repeat.

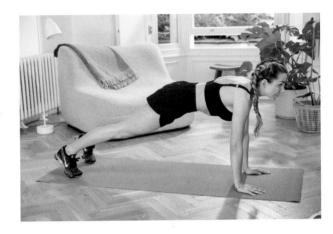

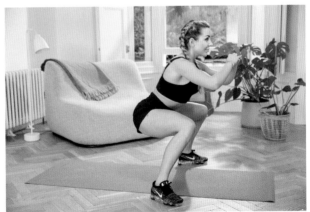

SQUAT OBLIQUE CRUNCHES

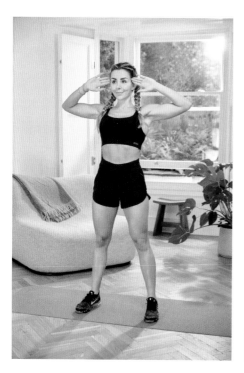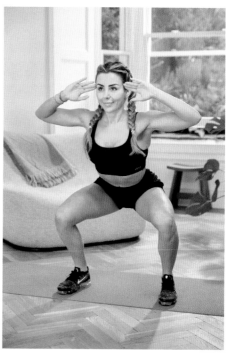

Start in standing position with your feet shoulder-width apart and arms by your head. Squat down, and as you stand up raise your right knee and meet it with your opposite elbow. Repeat, switching sides each time.

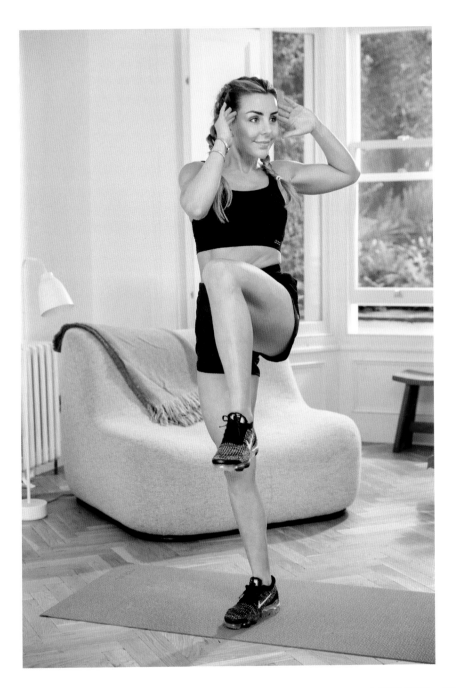

1½ SQUAT JUMPS

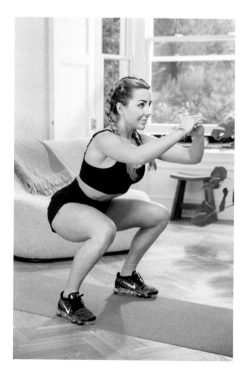
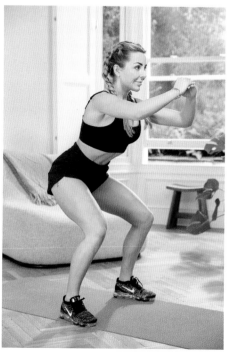

Start in standing position with your feet shoulder-width apart and bend into a squat position with your arms in front of your chest. Come halfway up before going back down into the squat, then jump into the air, pushing your arms behind you. Land back in the squat position. Make sure you do not bring your knees in. Repeat.

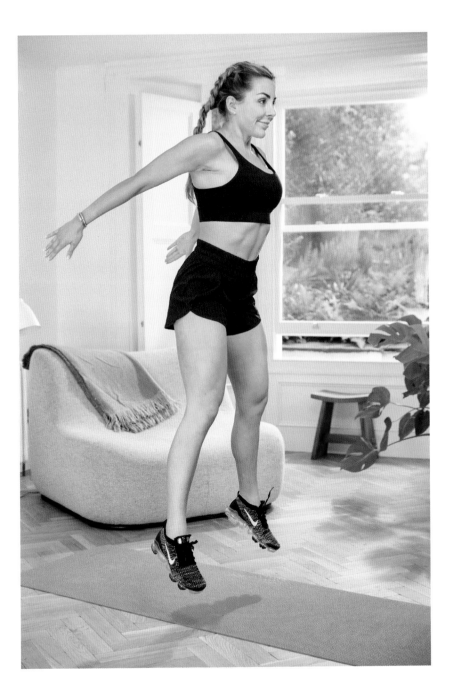

SKATER LUNGES

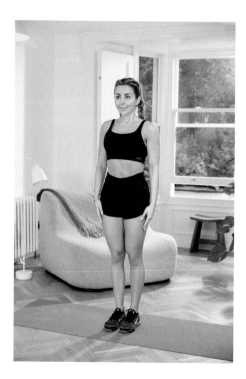
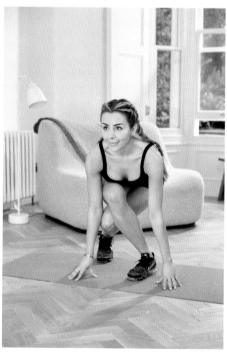

Start in standing position, arms by your side, then step your left foot behind your right leg (it should touch the floor) and bend both knees to lower into a lunge with your left knee behind your right heel and fingers touching the floor. Return to standing and repeat with the opposite leg at a fast pace.

BELT KICKS

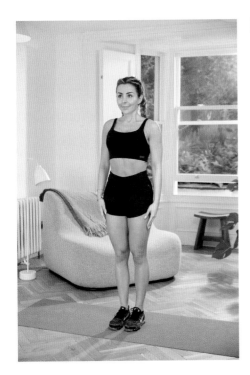 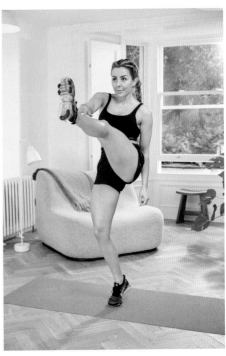

Start in standing position, legs together and arms by your side, then squat down and touch the floor. As you stand up, kick one leg out in front of you. Repeat, changing the legs in front of you each time.

STEP-BACK BURPEES

Start in standing position, then crouch down, putting your hands on the floor. Step your feet back into a high plank position. Return your feet back into a crouch by stepping them towards your hands. Stand up and reach up high. Repeat.

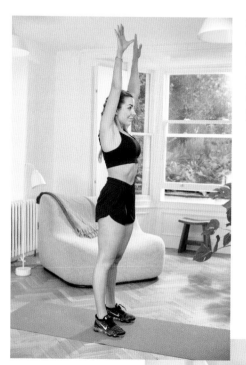

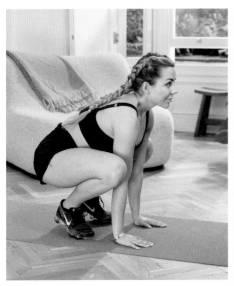

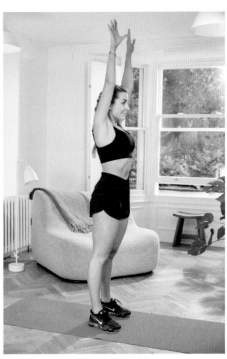

Push yourself, because no one else is going to do it for you

GROINERS

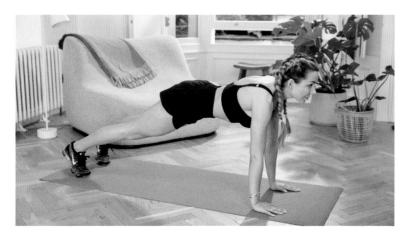

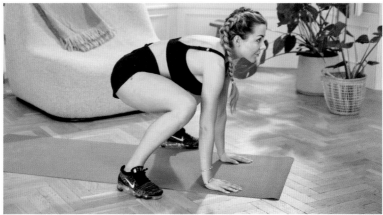

Start in a high plank position, then jump both your feet up towards your hands. Pause for a second, then jump back to a plank position.

PLANK JACKS

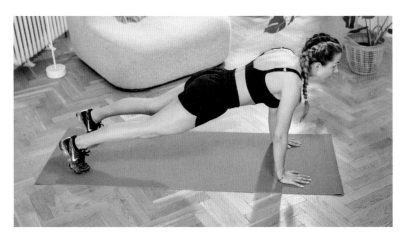

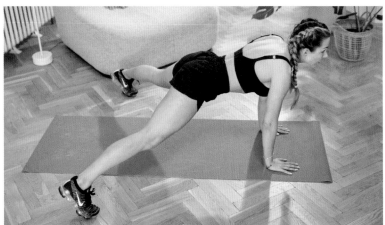

Start in a high plank position with your feet together. Jump your feet out and in, like you're in a horizontal jumping jack.

MOUNTAIN CLIMBERS

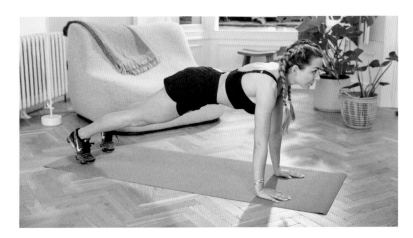

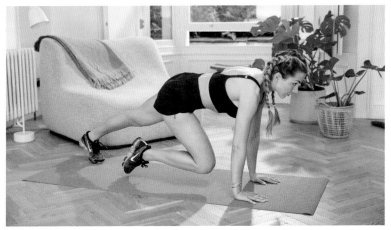

Start in a high plank position, with your core engaged and feet together. Draw your right knee towards your chest and then replace it. Do the same with your left knee, at a fast pace. Repeat.

CROSS CLIMBERS

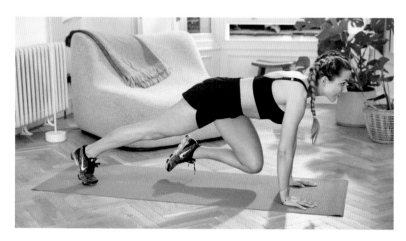

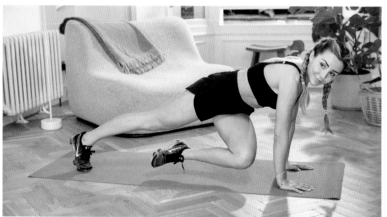

Start in a high plank position, with your core engaged and feet together. Draw your left knee in and across your body and then replace it. Do the same with your right knee, at a fast pace. Repeat.

ALTERNATE KNEE TAPS

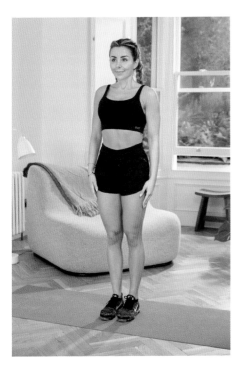 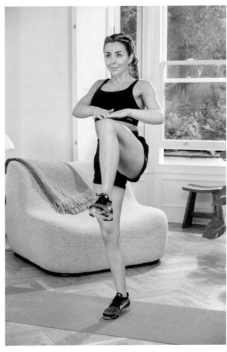

Start in standing position, arms by your side, and lift your left knee nice and high. Tap your hands onto your left knee. Do two quick jogs on the spot. Do the same with your right knee, moving at a fast pace. Repeat.

STAR JUMPS

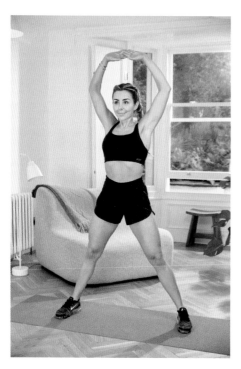 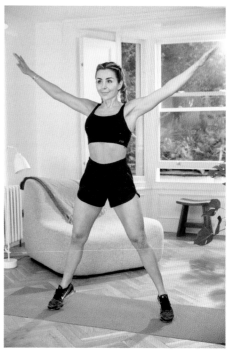

Start in standing position with your feet together and arms by your side. Jump your feet out to slightly further apart than your shoulders and simultaneously raise your arms above your head. Return to standing position, with feet together, and repeat.

SPRINT ON THE SPOT

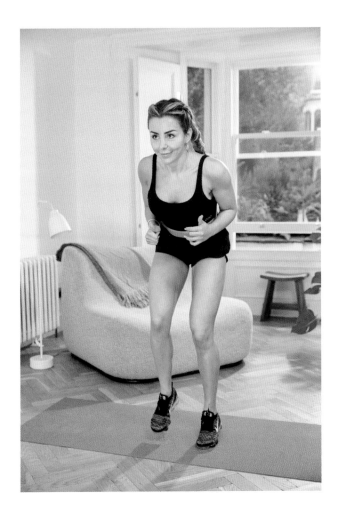

Run as quickly as you can on the spot.

HIGH KNEES

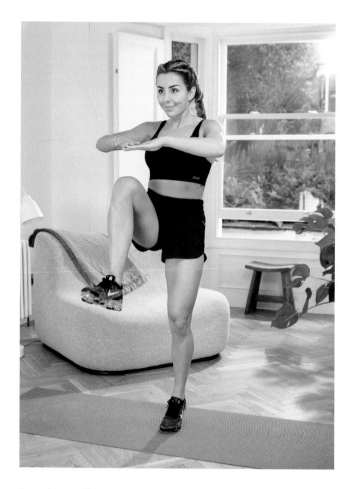

Start in standing position with your arms in front of your chest and raise your right knee to a 90-degree angle. Return your right foot to the ground and raise your left knee at the same time. Do it as fast as you can, so you get into a running motion.

KNEES

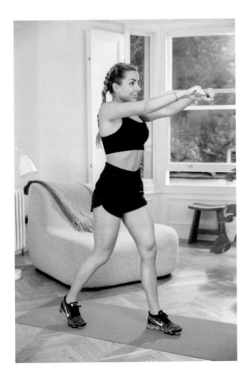 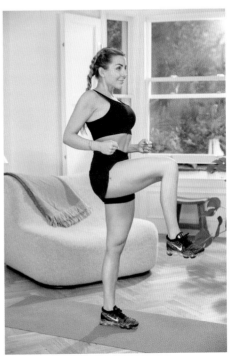

Take out your aggression by lifting your right knee as high as possible. Return your foot to the floor and repeat with your left leg.

BURPEES

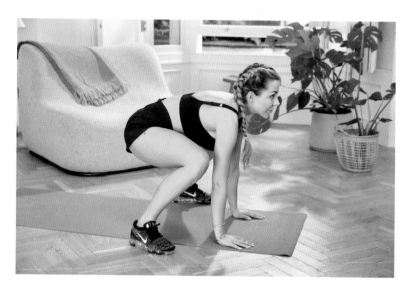

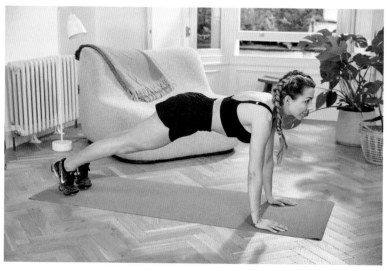

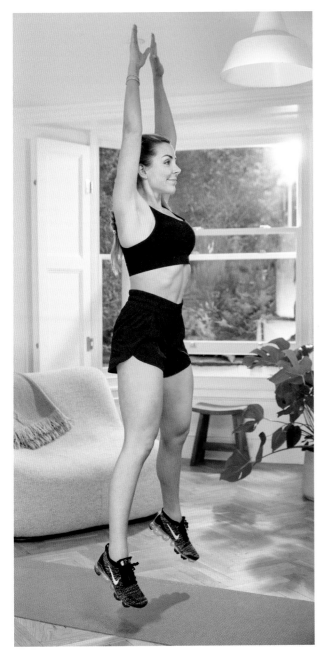

Start in standing position, then crouch down, putting your hands on the floor and legs wide. Jump your feet back into a high plank position. Return your feet back into a crouch, jumping them in between your hands. Stand up and reach up high, jumping off the floor. Repeat.

PUSH-BACK KNEE DRIVES

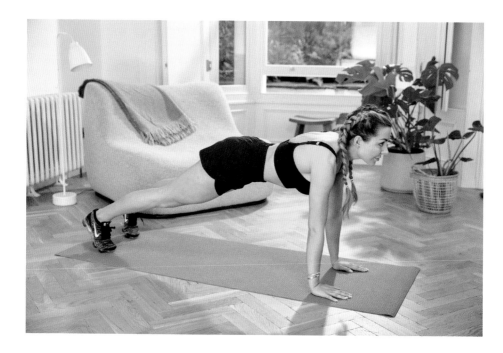

Start in a high plank position. Bend your knees and push your bodyweight back, bending your knees so your arms are stretched with your hands on the mat in front of you. As you push your weight back into your arms, drive your knees into your chest. Pause for a second, then jump your feet back to a plank position. Repeat.

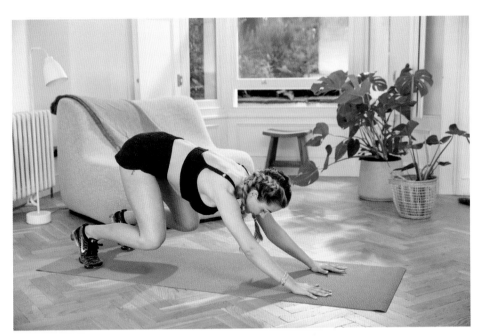

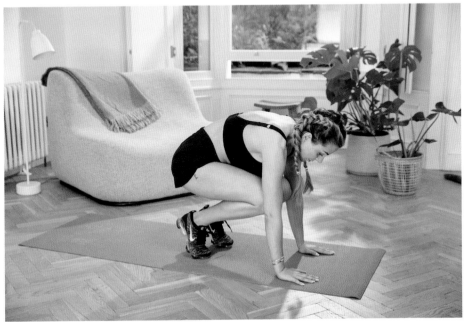

SNAP JUMPS

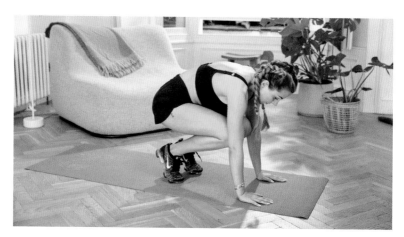

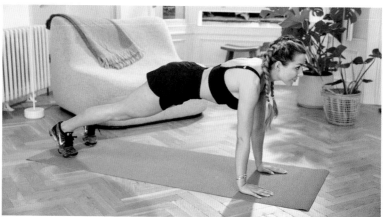

Start in standing position with both feet slightly wider than shoulder-width apart, bend your knees and place your hands on the floor in front of your feet. Jump both your feet backwards into a high plank position, then jump back towards your hands. Return to standing position and repeat.

SUICIDE DRILLS

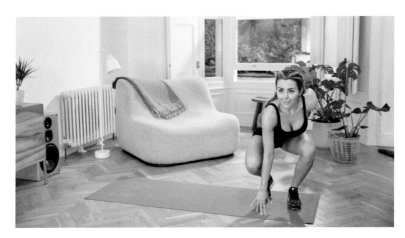

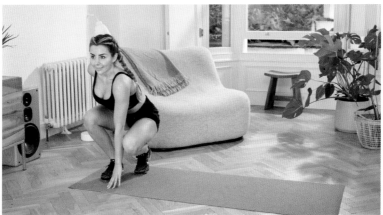

Start at one end of your mat and spring to the other end. Touch the floor with your hand and then spring back to the first point. Repeat.

CARDIO EXERCISES
TUCK JUMPS

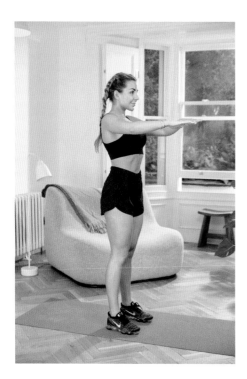
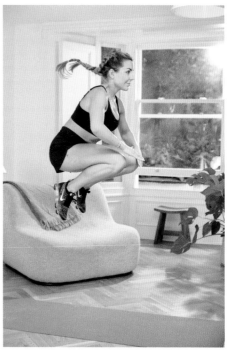

Start in standing position with your feet hip-width apart and your arms in front of your chest, then jump up as high as you can (really go for it, come on!) and grasp your shins with your hands as you bring your knees into your chest. Return to standing position and repeat.

FAST AIR PUNCHES

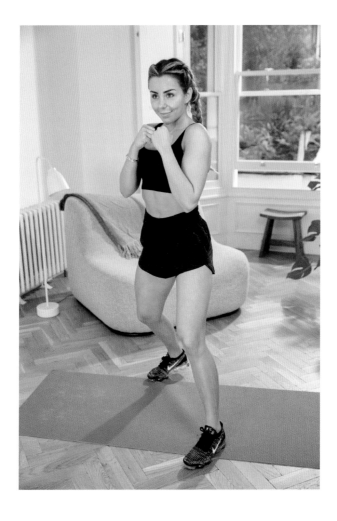

Let off some steam by punching your arms out in front of you, one at a time. Make sure to fully extend each arm.

CARDIO EXERCISES
WALKOUTS

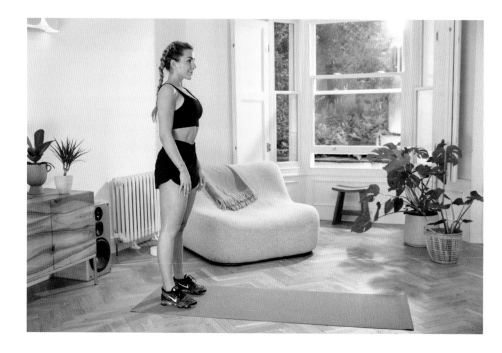

Start in standing position with your arms by your side, then hinge from the hips, reach your hands to the floor and walk your hands out until you are in a high plank position. Walk your hands back and stand up. Repeat.

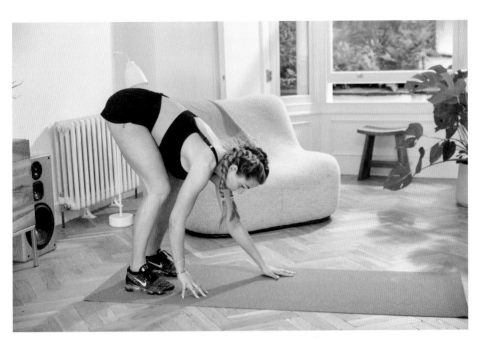

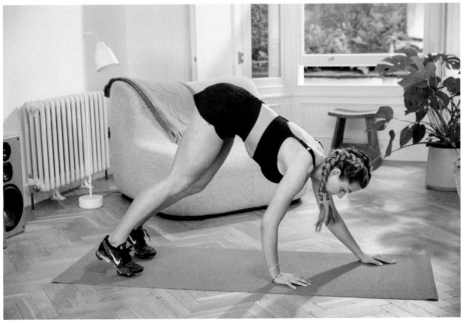

FULL-BODY EXERCISES

DUMBBELL SQUAT TO UPRIGHT ROWS

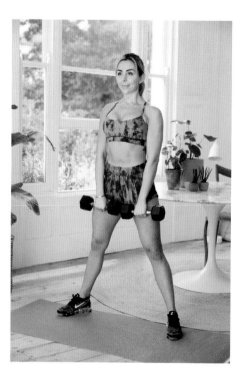
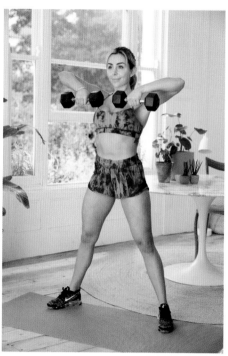

Start in standing position, with your feet wider than shoulder-width, and your arms straight down in between your legs, holding a dumbbell in each hand. Squat down, with your arms holding the dumbbells, and as you come up from the squat lift your elbows and row your arms up to shoulder level. Make sure you don't lift your shoulders up to your ears – keep them nice and relaxed.

DUMBBELL SQUAT PRESSES

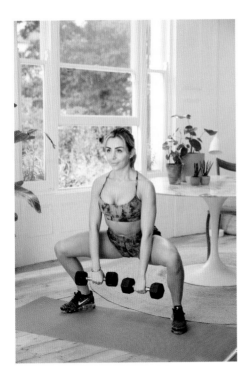
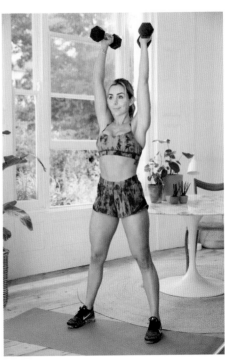

Start in standing position, with your feet wider than shoulder width, and a dumbbell in each hand. Rest the dumbells on your shoulders then squat down (until your thighs are parallel to the floor, if possible), keeping your core tight and your chest up. As you come up from the squat, still keeping your core tight, press the dumbbells above your head until your arms are straight, palms facing in, then lower the dumbbells with control. Repeat.

REVERSE-LUNGE BICEP CURLS WITH DUMBBELLS

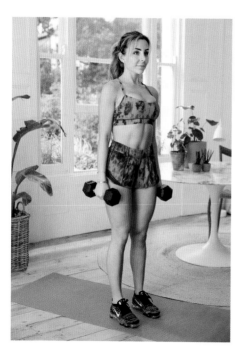
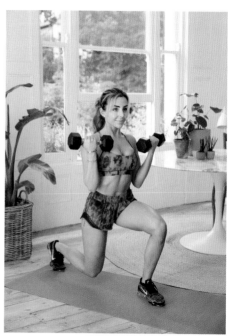

Start in standing position with a dumbbell in each hand, arms by your side, palms facing towards you and feet together. Take a large step back with one foot, and as you step back into a lunge (touching the floor with just the ball of your foot) lower your back knee towards the ground, keeping your core engaged and chest up, and curl your biceps up. Return to start position by driving through your heels and squeezing your glutes before alternating legs. Alternate legs each time you lunge back.

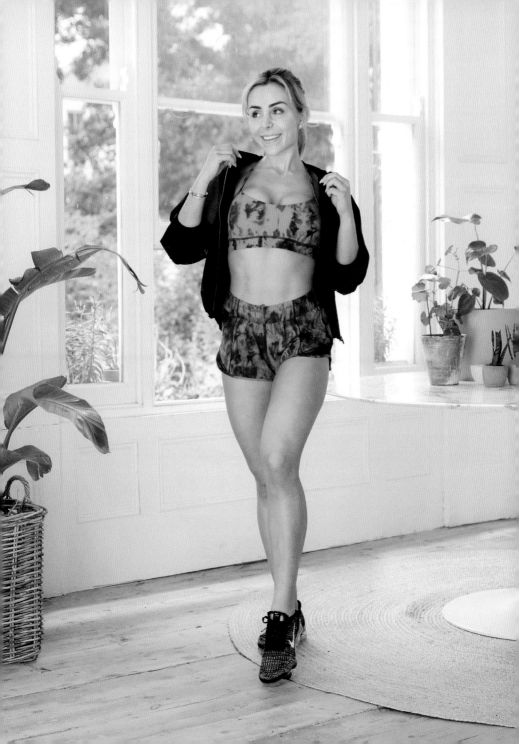

DEADLIFT INTO SHOULDER PRESS

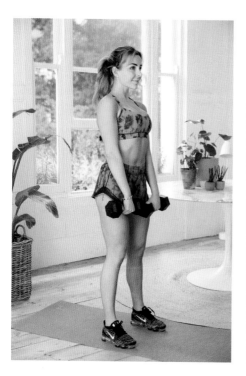
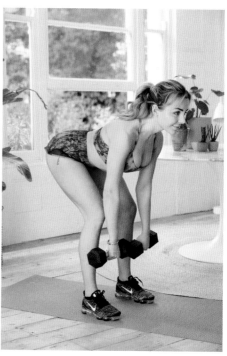

Pick up two dumbbells – choose your lighter weights. Start in standing position, with your feet shoulder-width apart and your hands holding the dumbbells in front of your legs with palms facing your body. As you bend your knees and lower down, brace your arms, keep your chest up and your core engaged. As you come back up, use your legs and core to lift the weights back up to standing position. Perform a conventional deadlift by shifting the weight to your collar bone and taking the dumbbells to a shoulder press. Bend your elbows to lower the weight back down.

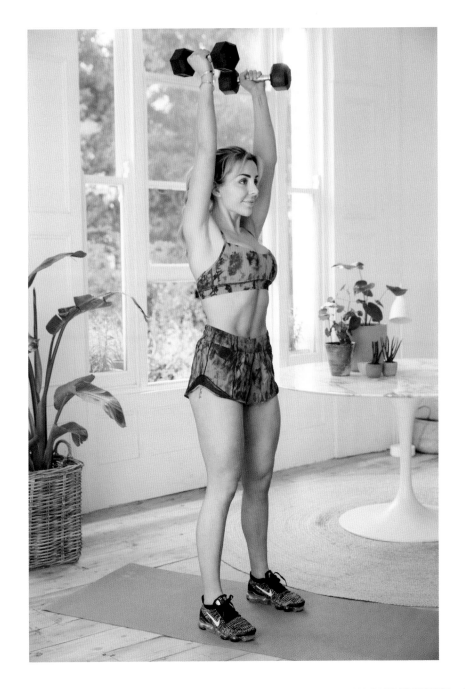

BURPEE RENEGADE ROW PRESSES

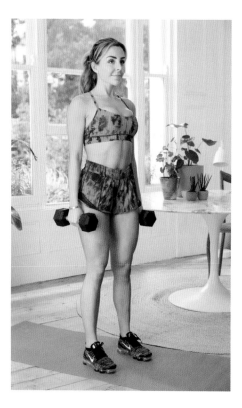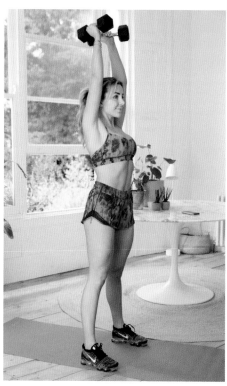

Start in standing position with a dumbbell in each hand and arms by your side, palms facing your body, then lower the dumbbells to the floor and burpee back (jump your legs back). Keep your core engaged and as soon as you are in the high plank position, one arm at a time, pull one dumbbell up towards your chest, bending at the elbow, then lower it down and do the same with the other dumbbell. As you row your arm up, squeeze your lats. As you lift the weights and stand up from the plank position, jump back into burpee/high plank position and row press on each side. Jump your feet back into crouch position, then stand up while pushing weights into a shoulder press. Bring weights down with control and repeat.

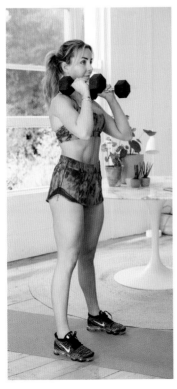

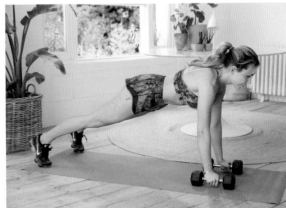

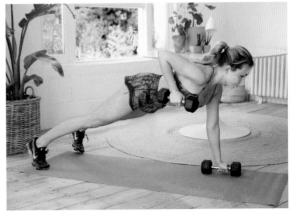

WEIGHTED BURPEE INTO SHOULDER PRESS

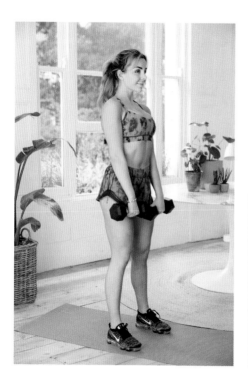
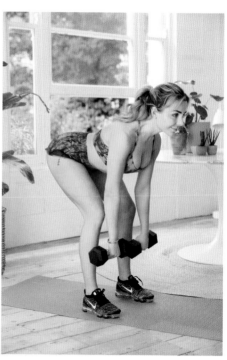

Start in standing position, feet shoulder-width apart, with a dumbbell in each hand and arms in front of your legs, palms facing in. Lower the dumbbells to the floor, squat and burpee back into high plank position, keeping your core tight. Stand back up to restart, bringing the weights with you (make sure you keep your back straight and chest up).

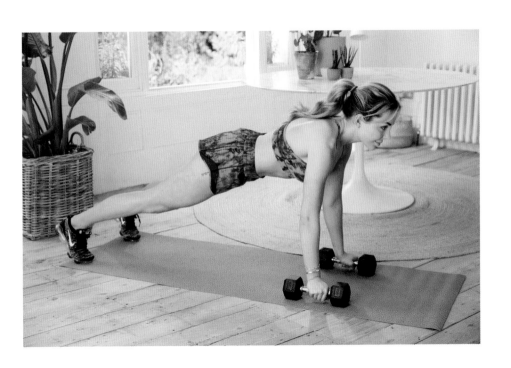

THE PLAN

WEEK ONE – THE WARM-UP

Okay, everyone, we're here! This is the start of your fitness journey with me, and I can't wait until you see how much fitter you are at the end of this week. The most important thing to remember this week is to take everything at your own pace. It's okay to be a beginner. Remember my mantra – we all start from somewhere. This is an amazing step for you, you're starting on your journey to feeling fitter and stronger. Don't forget to take your photos or measurements – whatever you're doing to see where you are right now and how much you're gonna improve over the next few weeks. You're at the start, and I'm here with you. The next 30 minutes are going to fly by and you're going to feel 10 times better once you've done this workout. Let's get sweaty!

DAY 1 – MONDAY
30-MINUTE HIIT CIRCUIT

 BREAKDOWN: Today we'll start with three HIIT circuits – you'll repeat each circuit once after you've done all five exercises. So, in total you'll do 30 rounds of exercises.

 TIMING: Do each exercise for 30 seconds and rest for 20 seconds before moving on to the next.

WARM UP

CIRCUIT 1:
1. SQUAT JUMPS
2. MOUNTAIN CLIMBERS
3. ALTERNATE KNEE TAPS
4. RUSSIAN TWISTS
5. STAR JUMPS

CIRCUIT 2:
1. SPRINT ON THE SPOT
2. SQUAT THRUSTERS
3. REVERSE-LUNGE LEG DRIVES
4. JUMP LUNGES
5. WALKOUTS

CIRCUIT 3:
1. HIGH KNEES
2. FAST AIR PUNCHES
3. CROSS CLIMBERS
4. BODYWEIGHT SQUATS
5. STEP-BACK BURPEES

COOL DOWN

DAY 2 – TUESDAY
FULL-BODY STRENGTH WORKOUT

BREAKDOWN: This is a full-body session, so make sure you have your dumbbells with you today. This is great for all-over toning, fat loss and burning loads of calories as you're hitting lots of muscle combinations here. There are five sets of exercises in total.

TIMING: Make sure you repeat all the reps per set before you move on to the next exercise. After each set rest for 45 seconds before moving on to the next.

WARM UP
1. SQUAT TO UPRIGHT ROWS: 3 SETS of 12 REPS
2. SQUAT PRESSES: 3 SETS of 12 REPS
3. BICEP CURLS INTO SHOULDER PRESSES: 3 SETS of 12 REPS
4. LATERAL RAISES: 3 SETS of 12 REPS
5. GOBLET SQUATS: 3 SETS of 15 REPS

COOL DOWN

REST DAY 3 – WEDNESDAY

You're halfway through the week and you've already made huge positive changes just by finishing those two workouts. Well done! I know you might be feeling the pain right now – you might be struggling to get out of bed in the morning, your chest and arms could feel tight and you may be achy all over – but don't worry, this is totally normal. As long as you're following the form tips that are in the descriptions to each move, there's nothing to worry about. Have a hot bath!

Just don't let any discomfort put you off continuing. Remember how much better you feel after you've finished your workout – more awake, energised and happier! You've already done so brilliantly by getting going on this, so let's push on through to the end of the first week – you can do it!

DAY 4 – THURSDAY
30-MINUTE HIIT SESSION

BREAKDOWN: This is really similar in structure to Monday's session, so you'll get the hang of this pretty quick! It's three HIIT circuits, and you repeat each circuit once after you've done all five exercises.

TIMING: Do each exercise for 30 seconds and rest for 20 seconds before moving on to the next.

WARM UP

CIRCUIT 1:
1. SKATER LUNGES
2. MOUNTAIN CLIMBERS
3. BELT KICKS
4. SQUAT JACKS
5. BURPEES

CIRCUIT 2:
1. GROINERS
2. KNEES
3. SQUAT JUMPS
4. FAST AIR PUNCHES
5. WALKOUTS

CIRCUIT 3:
1. PLANK JACKS
2. SQUAT OBLIQUE CRUNCHES
3. BODYWEIGHT RENEGADE ROWS
4. SPRINT ON THE SPOT
5. COMMANDOS

COOL DOWN

DAY 5 – FRIDAY
FULL-BODY WORKOUT

BREAKDOWN: A fab all-over session to give all your muscle groups a workout!

TIMING: Make sure you repeat all the reps per set before you move on to the next exercise. After each set rest for 45 seconds before moving on to the next set.

WARM UP

1. REVERSE LUNGES: 3 SETS of 20 REPS
2. CURTSY LUNGES WITH BICEP CURLS: 3 SETS of 20 REPS (10 PER SIDE)
3. CRUNCHES: 3 SETS of 20 REPS
4. STRAIGHT-LEG DEADLIFTS: 3 SETS of 12 REPS
5. BICEP CURL TO SHOULDER PRESS: 3 SETS of 12 REPS

COOL DOWN

REST DAYS 6 + 7 – SATURDAY + SUNDAY

I am so proud of you for getting this far. This is the first week done and you have already ticked off so many positive achievements this week. Remember how you felt at the start of the week – probably wondering how you were going to get through it all. But you have. You've smashed it and I know that however hard it's been for you, you'll already be feeling so much better now! Remember – what doesn't challenge you, doesn't change you.

Don't forget to log your progress for the week – whether that's measurements, improvement on reps or taking your photos. There might not be much change just now, but don't worry, you're just at the start of the journey.

Enjoy your rest days and use them as an opportunity to be nice to yourself. Treat yourself to a facemask, family time, a massage, a trip out with friends – anything that makes you feel really good and raring to go for Monday!

WEEK TWO - WARRIOR IN THE MAKING

Here we go, gang, into week two! Remember how you felt on day one just one week ago, and how much fitter you feel now on day eight … that's only going to improve again this week. Write down how you feel, so you remember how your mindset is changing. Perhaps you feel better each morning. Maybe you're sleeping better each night. It could be you've just got more energy overall and you can feel it. Every week you're going to see such amazing changes in your fitness levels. Stick with me: as your trainer I can tell you that you've got this, I promise you. I'm with you every step of the way.

There might be points this week that you find harder than last week. That's totally okay. Just don't give up. You can do this – you are a warrior. Let's go!

DAY 8 – MONDAY
HIIT AND ABS

 BREAKDOWN: Okay, guys, this is just like before – three HIIT circuits, and you repeat each circuit after all five exercises. Then there's an abs finisher at the end to tone up your tummy.

 TIMING: Do each exercise for 30 seconds and active rest for 10 seconds (light jog on the spot) before moving on to the next. You might not believe me right now, but active rest rather than actually stopping in between exercises actually makes it easier to carry on …

WARM UP

CIRCUIT 1:
1. 1½ SQUAT JUMPS
2. BURPEES
3. STAR JUMPS
4. MOUNTAIN CLIMBERS
5. PUSH-BACK KNEE DRIVES

CIRCUIT 2:
1. SNAP JUMPS
2. SUICIDE DRILLS
3. HIGH KNEES
4. GROINERS
5. POWER SQUATS

CIRCUIT 3:
1. JUMP LUNGES
2. FAST AIR PUNCHES
3. BELT KICKS
4. WALKOUTS
5. JUMP SQUATS

ABS FINISHER:
SIT-UPS:
2 SETS of 12–15 REPS
LEG RAISES:
2 SETS of 12–15 REPS

COOL DOWN

DAY 9 – TUESDAY
LEGS BLITZ

BREAKDOWN: This workout is focused on building strength in your legs. I'm gonna talk about 'super-sets' a couple of times today. These are exercises performed back to back with no rest in between – you rest after you've completed them both.

TIMING: Rest for 30 seconds between sets or super-sets.

WARM UP

1. GOBLET SQUATS: 3 SETS of 15 REPS

SUPER-SET WITH
2. SQUAT JUMPS: 3 SETS of 15 REPS
3. STRAIGHT-LEG DEADLIFTS: 3 SETS of 15 REPS
4. DUMBBELL REVERSE LUNGES: 3 SETS of 12 REPS PER LEG

SUPER-SET WITH
5. JUMP LUNGES: 3 SETS of 10 REPS PER LEG
6. DUMBBELL GLUTE BRIDGES: 3 SETS of 15 REPS
7. SQUAT JUMPS: 3 SETS of 20 REPS

COOL DOWN

DAY 10 – WEDNESDAY
UPPER-BODY FOCUS

BREAKDOWN: This session is going to really work out your arms, building strength and muscle tone.

TIMING: Rest for 30 seconds between sets or super-sets.

WARM UP

1. LYING CHEST PRESS: 3 SETS of 15 REPS
2. DUMBBELL UPRIGHT ROW: 3 SETS of 12 REPS

SUPER-SET WITH
3. DUMBBELL FLYES: 3 SETS of 12 REPS
4. BENT-OVER ROWS: 3 SETS of 15 REPS
5. BICEP CURLS INTO SHOULDER PRESSES: 3 SETS of 12 REPS
6. PRESS-UPS: 3 SETS of 10–15 REPS

COOL DOWN

REST DAY 11 – THURSDAY

Wow – we're into double-figure days and you're smashing it so far! I'm going to be honest, I've stepped it up a gear for you guys this week, and you've managed it like a pro! You're going to be giving me a run for my money soon.

Don't give up now, although I know this can be a tricky time. You can still feel a long way from 28 days, and maybe you feel as if you're not making enough progress. I promise you, however, that you are progressing, getting fitter, stronger and healthier with every minute more you invest in yourself, even if it doesn't feel like it right now. You might be considering skipping tomorrow's workout for an extra 30 minutes in bed or one last binge on your favourite TV programme – I get it. We all get tempted by the easy option sometimes, but listen to me, babes, get the workout done first and then reward yourself with telly, a bath or your bed! Self-discipline leads to success, and I promise you, if you prioritise your health and fitness, you will feel so much better for it, both inside AND out.

DON'T STOP
WHEN YOU'RE TIRED.
STOP WHEN
YOU'RE DONE.

DAY 12 – FRIDAY
HIIT AND ABS

 BREAKDOWN: It's our favourite circuit structure again – three HIIT circuits, and you repeat each circuit after all five exercises. After that there's the abs finisher.

 TIMING: Do each exercise for 30 seconds and active rest for 10 seconds (light jogging on the spot) before moving on to the next.

WARM UP

CIRCUIT 1:
1. BURPEES
2. SIT-UPS
3. WALKOUTS
4. SUICIDE DRILLS
5. GROINERS

CIRCUIT 2:
1. PUSH-BACK KNEE DRIVES
2. SQUAT JUMPS
3. BELT KICKS
4. MOUNTAIN CLIMBERS
5. STAR JUMPS

CIRCUIT 3:
1. POWER SQUATS
2. SNAP JUMPS
3. FAST AIR PUNCHES
4. SQUAT OBLIQUE CRUNCHES
5. CROSS CLIMBERS

ABS FINISHER:
PLANK HIP ROTATIONS:
2 SETS of 15 REPS PER SIDE
BICYCLE CRUNCHES:
2 SETS of 12 REPS PER SIDE

COOL DOWN

DAY 13 – SATURDAY
FULL-BODY WORKOUT

 BREAKDOWN: Another brilliant all-over session today that'll burn loads of calories. Six sets of exercises – and don't forget the super-set at the end.

 TIMING: After each set, rest for 45 seconds before moving on to the next set or exercise.

WARM UP

1. REVERSE-LUNGE BICEP CURLS: 3 SETS of 10 REPS PER LEG
2. BURPEE RENEGADE ROW PRESSES: 3 SETS of 10 REPS
3. SQUAT PRESSES: 3 SETS of 12 REPS
4. SQUAT TO UPRIGHT ROWS: 3 SETS of 15 REPS
5. LATERAL RAISES: 3 SETS of 12 REPS

SUPER-SET
6. PRESS-UPS: 3 SETS of 12–15 REPS

COOL DOWN

REST DAY 14 - SUNDAY

Yesss! Can you believe you're halfway through? Amazing work. You have to be super proud of yourself for getting this far – and make sure you let everyone around you know what you've achieved, too. You deserve some compliments and love, big time. I knew you could do it! Keep it up because this is just the beginning. You are making a positive lifestyle change and I am so happy for you! I want to make sure, too, that you're feeding yourself well at the moment, so spend a bit of time today cooking yourself something healthy and delicious. Food is your friend, and you'll need it more than ever at the moment!

Okay, so you know the drill: chart your progress today and see how far you've come. I bet by now you can see some really positive differences from where you were at the start of the plan. Whatever they are – well done!

I hope by now you feel like the workouts are becoming a part of your everyday life, and you're feeling the benefits. Because I promise you, your body and your mind are already in a better place than they were just a couple of weeks ago. Awesome work!

WEEK THREE – FIT, STRONG AND HEALTHY

Here we go, guys, it's week three! You're now closer to the end of the plan than the beginning – and you have come SO far. I know you're finding it tough right now, your body is probably aching more than usual, but trust me ... that's completely normal. Push through and be a warrior. To be a warrior you have to train like one.

Remember those goals you set back before you started the plan. Take a look back at them, read them, take your mind back to the place you were in when you wrote them. You could even add to them – write down how you're feeling now. Remember why you decided to start this journey to a healthier and happier you. Don't worry if you had a couple of slip-ups in the past couple of weeks, you're human. That's okay. The most important thing is to keep on going. You will thank yourself for it, I promise you. You can do this!

DAY 15 – MONDAY
FULL BODY AND HIIT

 BREAKDOWN: Today we've got one HIIT circuit for you to do, and you're gonna repeat it once after completing all eight exercises. After that you've got a strength finisher to burn out those muscles!

 TIMING: Do each exercise for 30 seconds and active rest for 10 seconds (light jog on the spot) before moving on to the next.

WARM UP

CIRCUIT 1
1. BURPEES
2. PUSH-BACK KNEE DRIVES
3. CROSS CLIMBERS
4. SQUAT JUMPS
5. SUICIDE DRILLS
6. JUMP LUNGES
7. POWER SQUATS
8. GROINERS

STRENGTH FINISHER:
SQUAT PRESSES: 3 SETS of 15 REPS
REVERSE-LUNGE BICEP CURLS:
3 SETS of 10 REPS PER LEG
SQUAT TO UPRIGHT ROWS: 3 SETS of 15 REPS
SUPER-SET WITH PRESS-UPS: 3 SETS of 15 REPS
RENEGADE ROW WITH DUMBBELLS: 3 SETS of 20 REPS

COOL DOWN

DAY 16 – TUESDAY
LEGS AND HIIT

BREAKDOWN: Same format as yesterday, guys! One HIIT circuit, which you repeat once after completing all eight exercises. Then a short legs session to finish off.

TIMING: Do each exercise for 30 seconds and active rest for 10 seconds (light jog on the spot) before moving on to the next.

WARM UP

1. SQUAT JUMPS
2. SNAP JUMPS
3. MOUNTAIN CLIMBERS
4. STAR JUMPS
5. 1½ SQUAT JUMPS
6. FAST AIR PUNCHES
7. WALKOUTS
8. BELT KICKS

LEGS FINISHER:
GOBLET SQUATS: 3 SETS of 12 REPS
Take 3 seconds on the way down/lowering phase
REVERSE LUNGES WITH PULSES: 3 SETS of 10 REPS PER LEG
STRAIGHT-LEG DEADLIFTS: 3 SETS of 20 REPS
SUPER-SET
GLUTE BRIDGES: 3 SETS of 20 REPS
SQUAT JUMPS: 3 SETS of 25 REPS

COOL DOWN

DAY 17 – WEDNESDAY
FULL-BODY WORKOUT

BREAKDOWN: It's back to the original HIIT style today, guys. Three HIIT circuits, and you repeat each circuit after all five exercises.

TIMING: Do each exercise for 20 seconds and rest for 10 seconds before moving on to the next. This is a fast-paced workout!

WARM UP

CIRCUIT 1:
1. STAR JUMPS
2. HIGH KNEES
3. SQUAT JUMPS
4. MOUNTAIN CLIMBERS
5. BURPEES

CIRCUIT 2:
1. WALKOUTS
2. GROINERS
3. SUICIDE DRILLS
4. FAST AIR PUNCHES
5. SQUAT OBLIQUE CRUNCHES

CIRCUIT 3:
1. JUMP LUNGES
2. SNAP JUMPS
3. SQUAT JACKS
4. SKATER LUNGES
5. PUSH-BACK KNEE DRIVES

ABS FINISHER:
SIT-UP RUSSIAN TWISTS:
2 SETS of 15 REPS
TUCKS: 3 SETS of 20 REPS

COOL DOWN

REST DAY 18 – THURSDAY

Oh yeah, what a week so far! I'm not going easy on you, you can see that, right? I'm not gonna apologise, it's all for your own good! But you've made it past the midweek point, which is the biggest achievement, so don't stop now. End the week on a positive note. Think about how amazing you are going to feel when you have completed another week. Again, it's going back to the mantra that what doesn't challenge you doesn't change you. I know you can do it.

Look back at your week-one pictures and look how far you have come. Keep that vision in your head while you finish the week. Think back to how different your fitness levels were. I bet you can tell the difference right now. Things are only going to get even better for you, so let's keep those energy levels up!

DAY 19 – FRIDAY
UPPER BODY AND HIIT

BREAKDOWN: Okay, so today we've got just one HIIT circuit, but I want you to repeat it two times after doing all five exercises. There's lots of super-sets today – I know you can do it!

TIMING: Do each exercise for 30 seconds and active rest for 10 seconds (light jog on the spot) before moving on to the next.

WARM UP

CIRCUIT:
1. WALKOUTS
2. BURPEES
3. PRESS-UPS
4. SQUAT JACKS
5. HIGH KNEES

LATERAL RAISES: 3 SETS of 15 REPS
SUPER-SET
BENT-OVER ROWS: 3 SETS of 15 REPS
RENEGADE ROWS: 3 SETS of 20 REPS
SUPER-SET
SHOULDER PRESSES: 3 SETS of 15 REPS
CLOSE-GRIP DUMBBELL PRESSES: 3 SETS of 12 REPS
SUPER-SET
DUMBBELL TRICEPS EXTENSIONS: 3 SETS of 12 REPS

COOL DOWN

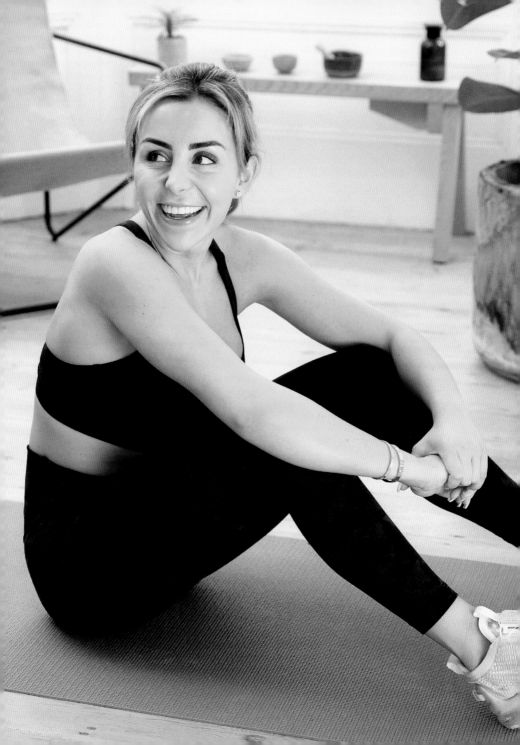

DAY 20 – SATURDAY
FULL-BODY AND ABS

 BREAKDOWN: Similar to yesterday, it's one circuit that I want you to repeat twice. We'll be working on your whole body today, and then finishing off with a focus on abs.

 TIMING: Do each exercise for 30 seconds and active rest for 10 seconds (light jog on the spot) before moving on to the next.

WARM UP

1. DEADLIFT INTO SHOULDER PRESSES: 3 SETS of 15 REPS
2. WEIGHTED BURPEE INTO SHOULDER PRESSES: 2 SETS of 12 REPS
3. BURPEE RENEGADE ROW PRESSES: 2 SETS of 12 REPS
4. V-UPS: 3 SETS of 10–20 REPS
5. SIT-UPS: 3 SETS of 12–20 REPS
6. SQUAT PRESSES: 3 SETS of 15 REPS

COOL DOWN

REST DAY 21 - SUNDAY

Phew! Three weeks in, that's actually incredible. It really is! You're three-quarters of the way through, the end is in sight now. You've made me proud. You have one week left of my plan, but remember, you've now formed a fantastic exercise habit, so it's not over once you reach the end of the four weeks. It's been said that it takes 21 days to create a new habit, so you've done it already, you've shifted to a more positive ritual.

Fitness isn't a quick fix, it's a lifestyle change. Keeping these 30-minute workouts in your day is going to change your life for the long run. Today, you need to do a couple of things. Firstly, chart your progress with those measurements, reps or pictures. Also, write down how you're feeling today, and don't forget to give yourself the credit you deserve. Remember the affirmations that you created for yourself? Now's the time to remind yourself of the ones that mean the most, because you are totally fulfilling them.

WEEK FOUR – THE FINAL BATTLE

How are you feeling? Aching? Energised? Excited? You're going to feel a mix of emotions this week, but that's normal. This is the week I want you to give every single workout 150 per cent effort ... no excuses. Let's end this challenge on a high!

Take a moment before you start Monday's workout to think about how far you've come. When you started this plan three weeks ago, I bet this point felt a million miles away. You might have felt that you couldn't do it – but you HAVE. That's fantastic. There have been sacrifices, there have been days where you probably wanted to collapse on the sofa rather than do another workout – but YOU DID IT. Self-discipline has led to success. And now look at how you feel, how your confidence has improved, how much fitter you are, how much healthier you feel. We're nearly there!

DAY 22 – MONDAY
LEG DAY

 BREAKDOWN: Today we've got three leg circuits. Each circuit you repeat once after all four exercises are done – making a total of 24 exercises in all.

 TIMING: Do each exercise for 45 seconds and rest for 30 seconds before moving on to the next.

WARM UP

CIRCUIT 1
1. GOBLET SQUATS
2. SQUAT JUMPS
3. STRAIGHT-LEG DEADLIFTS
4. SQUAT PRESSES

CIRCUIT 2
1. CURTSY LUNGES
2. GLUTE BRIDGES
3. POWER SQUATS
4. REVERSE LUNGES

CIRCUIT 3
1. LATERAL LUNGES
2. SPLIT SQUATS
3. JUMP LUNGES
4. REVERSE LUNGE WITH KNEE DRIVES

COOL DOWN

DAY 23 – TUESDAY
UPPER-BODY SESSION

BREAKDOWN: This is the same format as yesterday, but this time focusing on your arms and upper body. Three upper-body circuits; each circuit you repeat once after all four exercises are done, so a total of 24 again.

TIMING: Do each exercise for 45 seconds and rest for 30 seconds before moving on to the next.

WARM UP

CIRCUIT 1
1. RENEGADE ROWS
2. WALKOUTS
3. SHOULDER PRESSES
4. PRESS-UPS

CIRCUIT 2
1. BENT-OVER ROWS
2. BURPEES
3. DUMBBELL FLYES
4. MOUNTAIN CLIMBERS

CIRCUIT 3
1. SQUAT PRESSES
2. CROSS CLIMBERS
3. BICEP CURL INTO SHOULDER PRESSES
4. LYING CHEST PRESSES

COOL DOWN

DAY 24 – WEDNESDAY
FULL-BODY WORKOUT

BREAKDOWN: Can you see the theme building here?! Same format as Monday and Tuesday – three full-body circuits; each circuit you repeat once after all four exercises – but we're going to work your whole body today.

TIMING: Do each exercise for 45 seconds and rest for 30 seconds before moving on to the next.

WARM UP

CIRCUIT 1
1. BURPEE RENEGADE ROW PRESSES
2. DEADLIFT INTO SHOULDER PRESSES
3. HIGH KNEES
4. RENEGADE ROWS

CIRCUIT 2
1. SQUAT TO UPRIGHT ROWS
2. PRESS-UPS
3. REVERSE-LUNGE BICEP CURLS
4. SQUAT JUMPS

CIRCUIT 3
1. SQUAT OBLIQUE CRUNCHES
2. LYING CHEST PRESSES
3. WALKOUTS
4. GOBLET SQUATS

COOL DOWN

REST DAY 25 - THURSDAY

Wow – can you feel that finish line? Can you see it? You can almost touch it, you're so close! You need to pat yourself on the back, honestly, you've done me so proud. Enjoy your rest day today 'cause it's not over yet. Two workouts left this week and I have made them really high intensity … Ready? Let's go!

DAY 26 – FRIDAY
HIIT AND ABS

BREAKDOWN: Right – today's session is three HIIT body circuits. Each circuit you repeat once after all five exercises. You know the drill!

TIMING: Do each exercise for 30 seconds and go crazy – I want full intensity! Rest for 10 seconds before moving on to the next.

WARM UP

CIRCUIT 1:
1. TUCK JUMPS
2. MOUNTAIN CLIMBERS
3. SQUAT DROPS
4. BURPEES
5. BELT KICKS

CIRCUIT 2:
1. SQUAT JACKS
2. HIGH KNEES
3. PUSH-BACK KNEE DRIVES
4. STAR JUMPS
5. CROSS CLIMBERS

CIRCUIT 3:
1. WEIGHTED BURPEES
2. SNAP JUMPS
3. SQUAT PRESSES
4. GROINERS
5. SUICIDE DRILLS

ABS FINISHER:
SIT-UPS: 1 SET of 20 REPS
AB TUCKS: 1 SET of 20 REPS
BICYCLE CRUNCHES: 1 SET of 20 REPS
LEG RAISES: 1 SET of 20 REPS

COOL DOWN

DAY 27 – SATURDAY
HIIT AND ABS

BREAKDOWN: We're feeling the same vibes as yesterday – it's a full-on, high-intensity circuit training sesh! Three HIIT body circuits; each circuit you repeat once after all five exercises. It's your last one, so pull out all the stops and really go for it!

TIMING: Do each exercise for 30 seconds and rest for 10 seconds before moving on to the next.

WARM UP

CIRCUIT 1:
1. 10 HIGH KNEES INTO 2 BURPEES
2. WALKOUTS
3. TUCK JUMPS
4. 2 BURPEES INTO 10 MOUNTAIN CLIMBERS
5. SQUAT JUMPS

CIRCUIT 2:
1. SPRINT ON THE SPOT
2. SUICIDE DRILLS
3. CROSS CLIMBERS
4. SQUAT JACKS
5. SKATER LUNGES

CIRCUIT 3:
1. FAST AIR PUNCHES
2. SQUAT OBLIQUE CRUNCHES
3. SNAP JUMPS
4. BURPEES
5. PUSH-BACK KNEE DRIVES

ABS FINISHER:
V-UPS: 2 SETS of 10–20 REPS
REVERSE CRUNCHES: 2 SETS of 20 REPS
LEG RAISES: 2 SETS of 20 REPS

COOL DOWN

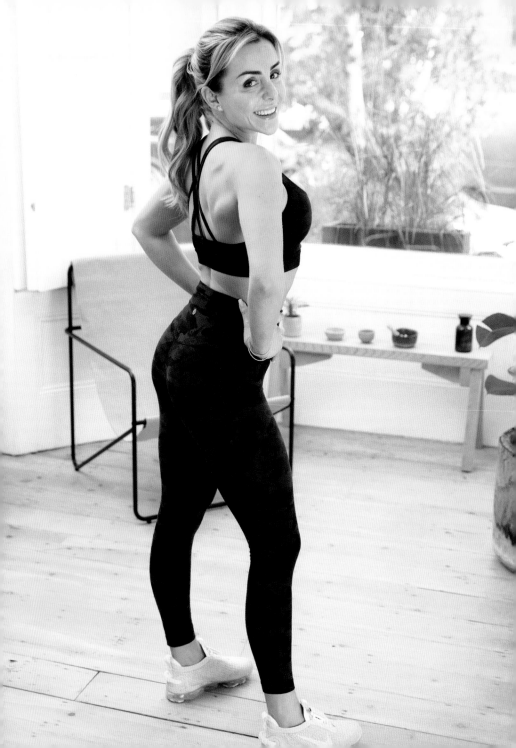

REST DAY 28 – SUNDAY

I AM SO PROUD!!! You have finished the plan and have made a fitter, healthier and happier version of yourself. Absolutely amazing – well done! This is such an achievement, you should feel brilliant about yourself right now.

You. Are. A. Warrior.

Take today to really reflect on the positive changes you've made. Go for a walk, a little jog, something that gives you the time and headspace to think about how this journey has been for you. Nothing too intense, just give yourself a little bit of me-time. When you get back home, look back at everything you wrote, photographed or measured on day one. Now's the time to appreciate just how far you've come and ask yourself the following questions …

How do you feel now overall?
What's your attitude to fitness now?
How has it changed?
What physical changes can you see in yourself?
Have you felt any mental and emotional changes?
What did you find the biggest challenge about this plan?
How did you overcome it?
What are you most proud of yourself for achieving?

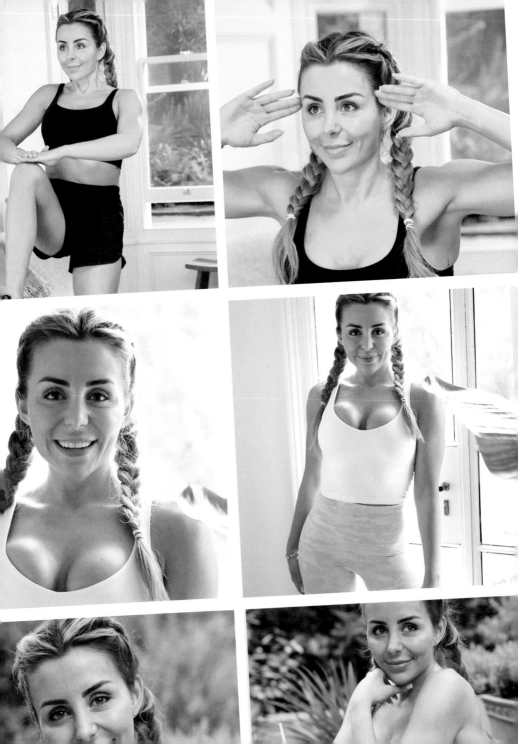

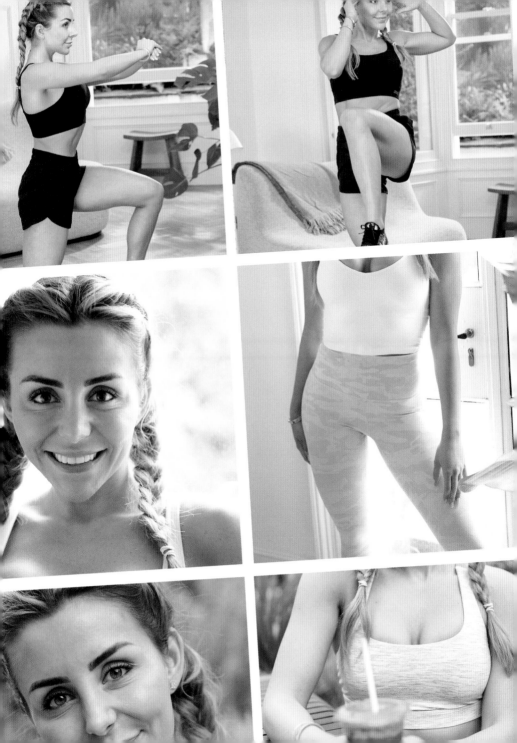

MOVING FORWARDS ...

Firstly, I want to say a huge THANK YOU to you for trusting in me as your Pocket PT. I hope that through this book you've been able to go on your own personal and powerful journey of transformation when it comes to fitness and mindset. You can see how much it's changed me over the years! I've shared my ups and downs with you, and how messed-up I was for a very long time when it came to my body and punishing myself. Nowadays, I still can't believe that was me. I've learned how to be a healthier, happier person, and honestly, now I feel the best I ever have. I've passed on all my life lessons to you, and hope that you can take them forward to help you become the best possible version of yourself.

You've completed the 28-day plan, which is an amazing achievement. But, this isn't the end! Remember that you've made this change for life now – you've made all the effort in finding the time every day, you've pushed yourself and done more than you ever thought you could. So don't drop it all now! This is your new way of living and it's so easy to keep it going.

'I DIDN'T GET THERE BY WISHING FOR IT, OR HOPING FOR IT, BUT BY WORKING FOR IT.'

ESTÉE LAUDER

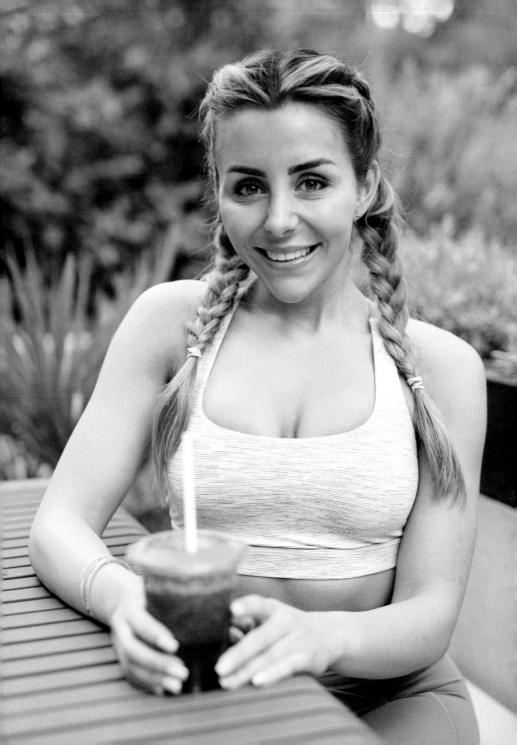

My app, Courtney Black Fitness, is the next tool you need to keep going with me as your trainer. You will have me with you every step of the way with your daily training, from home or the gym, and also your diet. I'll be in your pocket! You can follow along with me on my real-time workouts (like I'm there with you!) or follow a set plan like this one.

Whatever route you take now on your fitness journey, just know how proud I am of you – you have started this journey and changed your life. This is just the beginning.

Loads of love,

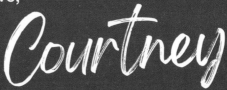

Courtney

ACKNOWLEDGEMENTS

Firstly, I'd like to thank the amazing, hardworking team at HarperCollins publishers: Helen, Oli, James and Sarah, and also Becky and Laura. You really listened to what I wanted for my book and brought the vision to life. To the shoot team who created the fantastic photos for the book – Sarah, Bella and David – thank you for being really accommodating, easy to work with, and for making me feel super comfortable.

Luke, my agent, was the person who suggested the idea of this book in the first place. I'd always wanted to do it, but never thought I'd be able to. Thanks, Luke, for being so supportive, believing in me and putting 100 per cent into everything.

Josh, my tutor in personal training and nutrition, was the person who put me on this path in my career. Thank you, Josh, for going above and beyond, putting in the extra hours and helping me.

Thanks to my best friend, Georgia, for always being so supportive.

My mum Colette has been there for me throughout all my struggles. She's worked so hard her whole life, and taught me how to work hard, too. Thanks for everything, Mum.

Finally, thank you so much to all the Instagram community and my followers. I really wouldn't be here if it wasn't for you all!

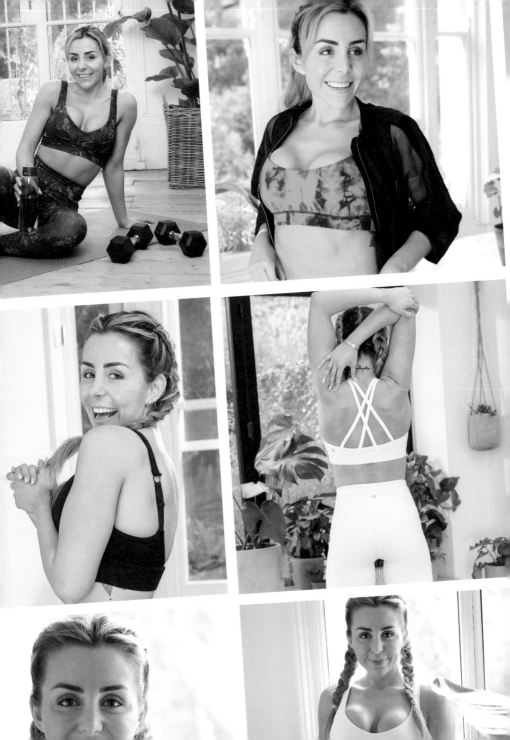